WEIGHT WATCHERS FREESTYLE 2018

By Anthony Young

The Ultimate Weight Watchers Freestyle Cookbook, The New Effective Way To Lose Fats! Enjoy Healthy, Tasty, & Clean Eating Recipes! **Plus Bundle Bonus!!**

Attention!!: This is a real bargain of 2 Manuscripts, (A two in one Book)

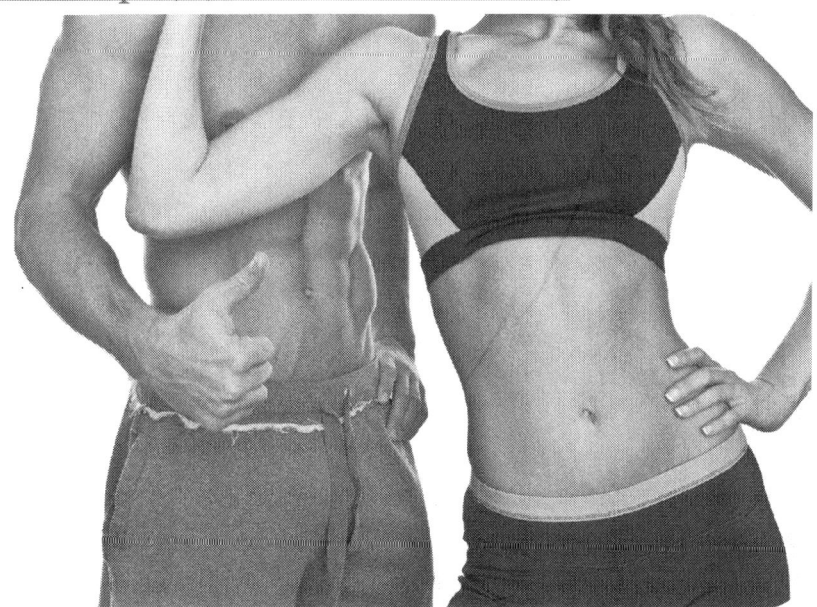

Book Number 1:

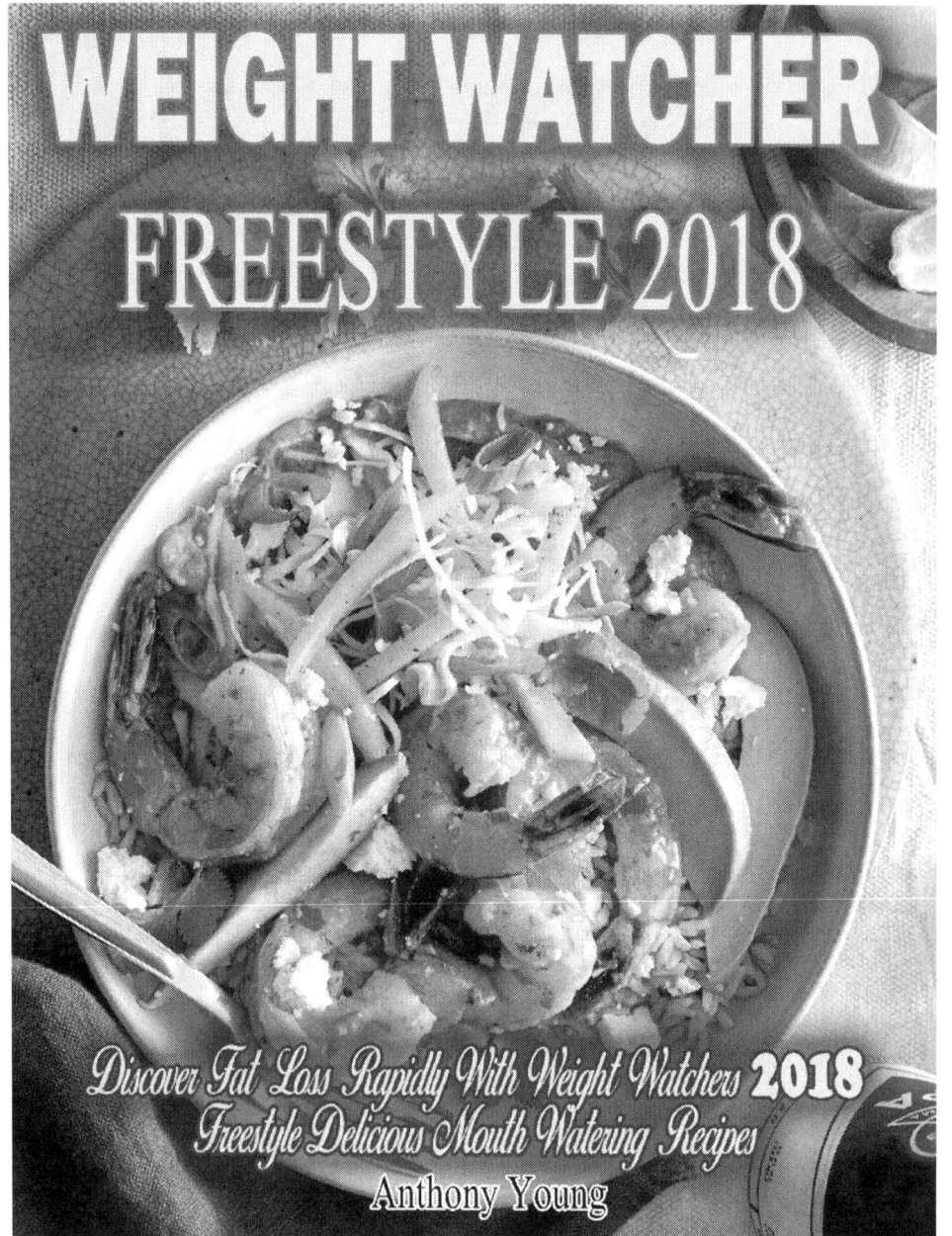

Book Number 2:

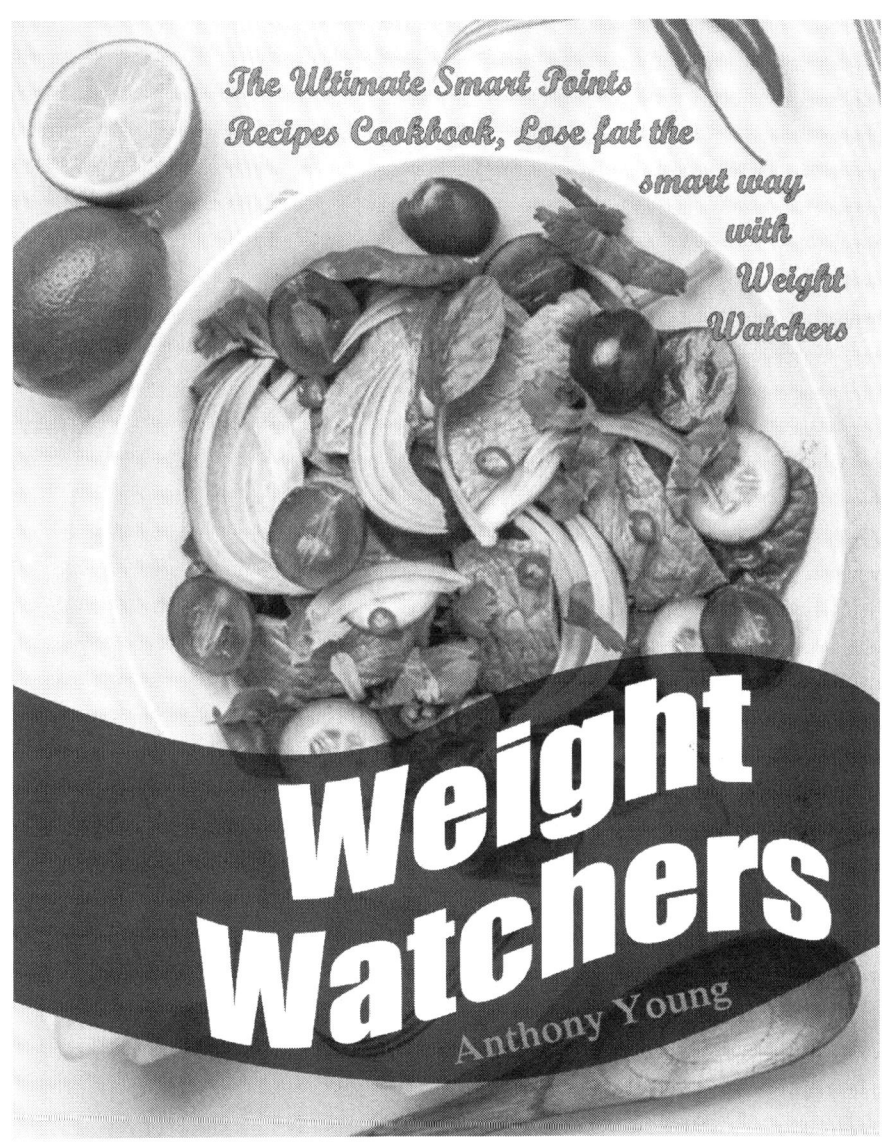

@ Copyright 2018 by Anthony Young All rights reserved.

In no way is it legal to reproduce, duplicate, or transmit any part of this document in either electronic means or in printed format. Recording of this publication is strictly prohibited and any storage of this document is not allowed unless with written permission from the publisher. All rights reserved.

The information provided herein is stated to be truthful and consistent, in that any liability, in terms of inattention or otherwise, by any usage or abuse of any policies, processes, or directions contained within is the solitary and utter responsibility of the recipient reader. Under no circumstances will any legal responsibility or blame be held against the publisher for any reparation, damages, or monetary loss due to the information herein, either directly or indirectly.

Respective authors own all copyrights not held by the publisher.

The information herein is offered for informational purposes solely, and is universal as so. The presentation of the information is without contract or any type of guarantee assurance.

The trademarks that are used are without any consent, and the publication of the trademark is without permission or backing by the trademark owner. All trademarks and brands within this book are for clarifying purposes only and are the owned by the owners themselves, not affiliated with this document.

Table of Contents

Book Number 1: 2
Book Number 2: 3
Introduction 9
LOOK AT HOW ZERO POINTS WORK: 11
EXAMPLES OF WEIGHT WATCHERS ZERO POINTS FOOD LIST: 13
    Limit these Food In Your Diet 19
    Include These Food In Your Diet: 20
WW FREESTYLE RECIPES 23
    Oregano Balsamic Chicken Lettuce Wraps 24
    Mushroom Ginger Chicken Soup 26
    Delicious Slow Cooker Chicken 27
    Yummy Vegetarian Chili 28
    Tasty Grilled Shrimp Kebabs 29
    Delicious Lime Asparagus Chicken 30
    Yummy Chicken Skewers 31
    Delicious Noodle Chicken Soup 32
    Oregano Cumin Chili Chicken 33
    Delight Marinated Chicken 34
    Chili Jalapeno Salsa Roasted Salmon 35
    Oregano Celery Turkey Chili 36
    Delicious Caramelized Garlic Pork Chops 37
    Yummy Grilled Chicken Nuggets 38
    Buffalo Chicken In A Slow Cooker 39
    Simple Salad Egg Sandwiches 40
    Tasty Pork Ragu 41
    Tasty Tenderly Chicken Baked 42
    Sunday Mouth-Watering Steak 43

Basil Sausage Cannellini Beans Soup 44
Chapter 3 Conclusion 45
Book Number 2 46
Introduction 47
Chapter 1: What is Weight Watchers? 49
    The Various Weight Watchers Plans 52
    What does it mean by 'Points'? 54
    What's good about Smart Points 56
    The Cons of Smart Points 57
    SmartPoints Values List: 59
    Why You Should Attend Meetings: 93
    Why You Should Get A Coach? 94
Chapter 2 Weight Watchers Breakfast Recipes 98
    Delicious Asparagus Pancetta Potato Hash 99
    Egg Avocado Toast in a Hole 100
    Yummy Lemon Poppy Seeds Muffins 101
    Onion Hash Browns Omelet 102
    Cheesy Tomato Ham Egg Bake 103
    Scallion Eggs Tomato Breakfast 104
    Cinnamon Pineapple Raisin Bread 105
    Healthy Breakfast Burrito 106
    Cinnamon Oatmeal Muffin with Applesauce 107
    Nutritious Avocado and Pear Smoothie 108
    Artichoke Spinach Breakfast Bake 109
    Hash Browns Bacon & Eggs 110
    Tasty Basil Zucchini Omelet 111
    Onion Tomato Avocado Scramble 112
    Simple Chia Pudding 113

Toasted Hazelnuts Apple & Chicken Omelette 114

Oregano Garlic Sweet Potato Spinach Casserole 115

Simple Cinnamon Oatmeal Muffin Breakfast 116

Basil Garlic Veggie-Egg Breakfast 117

Chapter 3 Weight Watchers Main Course Recipes 118

Parsley Garlic Eggplant "Meatballs" 119

Chili Cumin Grilled Steak 120

Delicious Beef Stew 121

Yummy Chili Garlic Thai Chicken 122

Delicious Broccoli Pineapple Pork 123

Onion Paprika Breaded Veal Cutlets 124

Asparagus Italian Steak Rolls 125

Garlic Dijon Chicken 126

Onion Leek Red Wine Steak 127

Cheddar Broccoli Chicken Noodle Casserole 128

Delicious Roasted Leg of Lamb 129

Jalapenos Garlic Macaroni Chili Turkey 130

Sesame Oregano Grilled Salmon Kebabs 131

Delight Chicken Stroganoff 132

Raisin Grilled Chicken Salad 132

Carrots Scallion Chicken Fried Rice 133

Cilantro Parsley Pork Chops with Salsa 134

Garlic Sweet & Sour Chicken 136

Weekend Treat Beef Burgundy 136

Tasty Turkey Cheeseburger & Broccoli Slaw 138

Coriander Jalapenos Sour Spicy Beef 139

Ginger Sesame Chicken 139

Tomato Lime Beef Curry 140

Chapter 4 Weight Watchers Seafood Recipes 141

Lemon Dijon Whitefish 142
Ginger Chili Salmon 142
Dill Coriander Cucumber Salmon 143
Cherry Tomato Asparagus Lobster Salad 144
Delicious Coconut Salmon 144
Spices Honey Shrimp Baked 145
Simple Tuna Salad 146
Ginger Honey Glazed Salmon 147
Spinach Tomato Shrimp Pasta 148
Yummy Tuna Salad & Pasta 149
Asian Style Sesame Glazed Salmon 150
Coconut Curry Scallops 151
Yummy Ginger Soy Sauce Salmon 152
Romaine Watermelon Salad & Shrimp 153
Parsley Garlic Pasta Shrimp 154

Chapter 5: Weight Watchers Desserts Recipes 155

Chocolate Cheesecake Cups 156
Raspberry Coconut Chia Pudding 157
Delicious Pumpkin Pudding 157
Walnut Dark Chocolate Clusters 158
Simple Truffles 158
Fruit Parfaits Candy Corn 159
Frozen Pineapple Berry Dessert 159
Vanilla Cranberry Coconut Macaroons 160
Nutmeg Pumpkin Cheesecake 161
Vanilla Cupcake Brownies 162
Raspberry Jam Banana Roll Ups 163

Chapter 5 Conclusion 163

Introduction

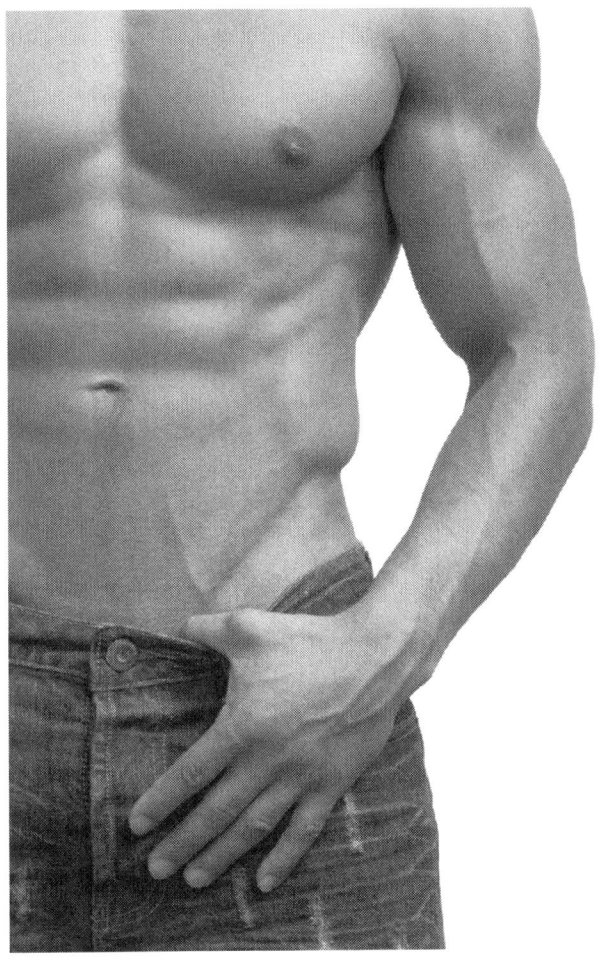

Congratulation and thank you for your purchase of my book, "*Weight Watchers Freestyle 2018:* **Discover Fat Loss Rapidly With Weight Watchers 2018 Freestyle Delicious Mouth-Watering Recipes!**

This book contains proven steps and strategies on how to lose weight, and maintaining your health.

The Weight Watchers weight loss program has gained a ton of popularity over the years due to its effective and easy techniques and methods to lose weight and keep at optimal health.

Of course, some of you have heard of Smart Points. And maybe Low Smart Points, and now get ready for Zero points! Make no mistake, this is the new way for Weight watchers. Weight Watchers Freestyle!
Join everyone in the newest trend for Weight Watchers. The Weight Watchers diet has been updated to its most optimal state as a Freestyle diet plan. Find out more about Zero points, and how this new measurement system is making all the difference. Weight Watchers Freestyle is the newest plan. Change is just around the corner, with new daily points goals, food, rollover points, and more.

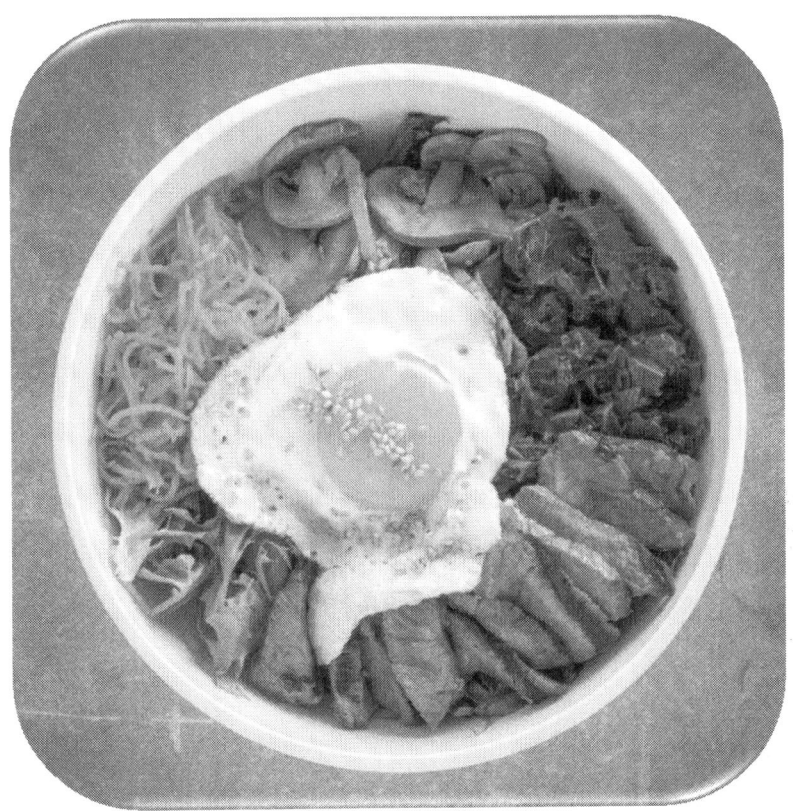

LOOK AT HOW ZERO POINTS WORK:

The biggest change to the diet plan is the new and innovative Zero Points. Although the old diet included fruits and veggies in adequate amounts, lean proteins are now added to the mix.

Various chicken types, such as skinless, lean ground and boneless chickens; skinless, thin sliced deli, lean ground, and boneless turkey; fresh seafoods, canned fish, tofu as well as eggs are now all foods classed as zero points.

Some foods have been reclassified based on their points. Non-dairy products such as yoghurt, soy yoghurt, as well as legumes are now worth nothing in Smartpoints values. Corn and Peas also were added to the Zero points values.

All Weight Watchers members will find this a welcome change, and the Zero points system is what many are most excited about. Legumes, fresh veggies, fresh fruits, as well as lean proteins are given a bigger focus in this new program structure. This continues to push members who are already using smartpoints to go even further, encouraging them to take up healthier choices and consume less foods that have a high degree of processing.

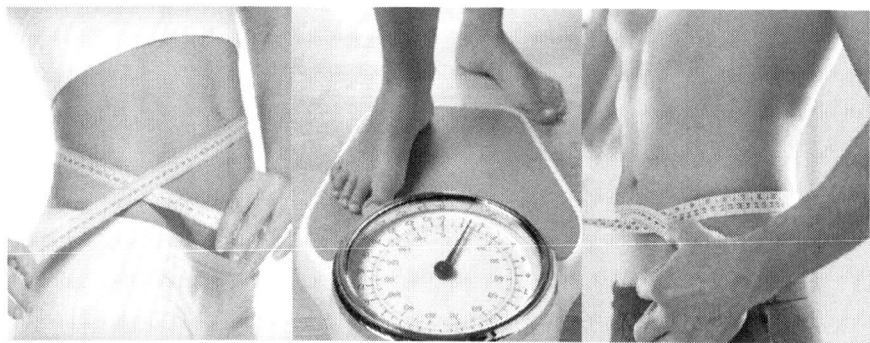

There are many programs that encourage dieting, but don't work as well compared with Zero points. Most will say the foods you can and can't eat, as well as the calories you ought to be taking in, including some restrictions intended to help, but are oftentimes frustrating to deal with. On the other hand if you use a points system, you don't have as many limits.

Your foods, your choice. There can be any number of food combinations you can eat, not restricting your diet pan to a few bland foods you'll bore of over time.

Weight watchers diet programs clinically supported to allow fast and effective weight loss, with the push towards uptake of healthy habits for better living. Don't listen to us, your body will feel the benefits soon enough!

EXAMPLES OF WEIGHT WATCHERS ZERO POINTS FOOD LIST:

- Apples
- Applesauce, unsweetened
- Artichokes
- Arugula
- Asparagus
- Apricots
- Arrowroot
- Artichoke hearts
- Bamboo shoots
- Banana

- Beans: cannellini, cranberry (Roman), green, garbanzo (chickpeas), kidney,

- lima, lupini, mung, navy, pink, pinto, small white, snap, soy, string, wax, white
- Beans, refried, fat-free, canned
- Broccoli slaw
- Broccolini
- Brussels sprouts

- Blackberries
- Blueberries
- Broccoli
- Broccoli rabe
- Beets
- Berries, mixed

- Cabbage: all varieties including bok choy, Japanese, green, red, napa, savory, pickled
- Cauliflower
- Caviar
- Celery
- Calamari, grilled
- Cantaloupe
- Carrots
- Swiss chard
- Cherries
- Chicken breast, ground chicken
- Chicken breast or tenderloin, skinless, boneless or with bone
- Clementines
- Coleslaw mix
- Collards
- Daikon
- Dates, fresh
- Eggplant
- Eggs, whole, including yolks
- Endive
- Escarole
- Dragon fruit
- Corn, baby corn

- Cranberries
- Cucumber
- Edamame, in pods or shelled
- Egg substitutes
- Egg whites
- Figs

- Fish: Almost all kind of fish

- Garlic
- Ginger root
- Grapefruit
- Grapes
- Greens: beet, collard, dandelion, kale, mustard, turnip
- Greens, mixed baby
- Guavas
- Guavas, strawberry

- Hearts of palm (palmetto)
- Honeydew melon
- Jackfruit
- Jerk chicken breast
- Artichokes

- Kiwifruit
- Kumquats
- Lime zest
- Lychees
- Mangoes

- Melon balls
- Mung bean sprouts
- Leeks
- Lemon
- Lemon zest
- Lentils
- Lettuce
- Lime
- Mung dal
- Mushroom caps
- Mushrooms: all kinds
- Nectarine
- Nori seaweed

- Peas and carrots
- Peas:all kinds
- Peppers, all varieties
- Pepperoncini
- Onions
- Oranges
- Papayas
- Parsley
- Passion fruit
- Pea shoots
- Peaches
- Peapods, black-eye
- Pears

- Persimmons
- Pickles, unsweetened

- Pico de gallo
- Pimientos, canned
- Pineapple
- Plums
- Pomegranate seeds
- Pomegranates

- Pumpkin
- Pumpkin puree
- Radicchio
- Radishes
- Raspberries
- Rutabagas

- Salad, mixed greens
- Salad, three-bean
- Salad, tossed, without dressing
- Salsa verde
- Salsa, fat free
- Salsa, fat free; gluten-free
- Sashimi
- Satay, chicken, without peanut sauce
- Satsuma mandarin
- Sauerkraut
- Scallions
- Seaweed
- Shallots

- Shellfish: abalone, clams, crab (including Alaska king, blue, dungeness, lump crabmeat, queen) crayfish, cuttlefish, lobster (including

- spiny lobster), mussels, octopus, oysters, scallops, shrimp, squid
- Spinach
- Sprouts, including alfalfa, bean, lentil
- Strawberries
- Succotash

- Tangelo
- Tangerine
- Taro
- Tofu, all varieties
- Tofu, smoked
- Tomatillos
- Tomato puree
- Tomato sauce
- Tomatoes: all varieties including plum, grape, cherry
- Turkey breast, ground, 99% fat-free
- Turkey breast or tenderloin, skinless, boneless or with bone
- Turkey breast, skinless, smoked
- Turnips

- Vegetable sticks
- Vegetables, mixed
- Vegetables, stir fry, without sauce

- Water chestnuts

- Watercress
- Watermelon

- Yogurt, Greek, plain, nonfat, unsweetened
- Yogurt, plain, nonfat, unsweetened
- Yogurt, soy, plain

Limit these Food In Your Diet

- Sugar is a cause of many diseases like diabetes and other heart ailments. Artificial sweeteners are also not a very healthy option even though they don't have calories.

- Grains can be quite fattening especially gluten grains like wheat and barley. Rice and oats are a healthier alternative.
- Trans-fat-containing foods are unhealthy and found in many processed foods.

- Foods labeled as "diet" or "low-fat" are not healthy either. They usually contain a lot of sugar and are quite processed.

- Processed foods, in general, are not a very healthy option. They contain harmful additives and have low nutritive value as well.

- Alcohol is also harmful to your body in general and can cause weight gain if excessively consumed in forms like beer. A glass of wine or two is not as harmful.

- Sodas and other sugary drinks actually contain a lot of sugar and many chemicals as well.

- Deep-fried food like chips and French fries are also bad for your body and contain a lot of calories.

- Ice cream and chocolates should be consumed in a controlled amount and not too frequently.

We don't recommend that you completely cut off these foods from your diet. If you especially like a certain food, it is even harder to stick to a diet that restricts you from having that food completely. This is why you should just be more conscious about how much you eat these foods without having to feel guilty about it later. As you become more conscious about what you eat, it will become a more natural initiative for you to choose the healthier option the next time you eat.

Include These Food In Your Diet:

- Eggs are a very nutritious option for you as long as you do not consume too many
- Meat is a healthy addition to your diet too. Please includes meat whenever possible. Fresh Lean Meat (Any kind is the way to go)
- Fish is one of the healthiest things to include in your diet. Fish contains many nutrients and healthy omega-3 fatty acids, it help your brain to work properly.
- Fruits (all kinds) should be included in your diet regularly, they contains vitamin C which also one of the most important thing that our body need every day.

- Vegetables is a must to includes in your daily meals, they provide your body lots of nutrients, if you want to gain the maximum benefits in your well-being
- Nuts and seeds, contains a lot of Vitamin E, but they're should be consumed in moderation because of their high-calorie content.

Carbohydrates: Even though when you are a diet, too much Carbs is not good, but they are still should be consumed in moderation but not completely restricted even if you are trying to lose weight. Once you are more aware of how different foods affect your body, you can make better choices. Healthy eating habits to incorporate into your daily life:

- Drink water. Cut out the habits of drinking alcohol or other sweet drinks, by introduce water intake more often and make as a routine of Drinking a glass of warm water with honey and lemon juice after you wake up every day, will do you even better

- Pay attention to your serving sizes during meals, especially the grains. Split dishes with a friend when you eat out. Avoid ordering large portions of anything because your body does not need it.
- Eat slowly and chew well after each bite in order to help digest your food well. Your brain then processes when you have had enough food. This does not happen on time when you gulp down food too fast.
- Eat a filling breakfast every single day without skipping.
- Eat small meals throughout the day instead of three large meals. This keeps your energy level up the whole day and also prevents binge eating due to hunger.

- Choose healthier cooking methods like grilling. When you stir fry your meat or veggies, use a few healthy oils like olive oil. Steaming vegetables is also good. Replace salt with herbs or spices.
- Eat dinner at least a couple of hours before you sleep.
- Do not eat large snacks after dinner.
- Include fiber in your meals in the form of whole grains, apple, berries, beans, vegetables, etc.
- Limit your salt intake. Keep note of the content especially in packaged foods, as they tend to be high in salt..
- Eat the actual fruit instead of opting for juices, especially processed juices. The fruit will benefit your body much more. They give you more fiber
- Choose lean meat and cut down on animal fat in your diet. Animal fat will increase bad cholesterol levels in your body.

- Consume calcium and vitamin D in your diet for bone health.
- Avoid alcohol or limit it to a glass or two a day if you must. Moderate amounts of wine or such might benefit you but the problems associated with too much alcohol suggest you avoid it altogether.

Weight Watchers Freestyle Recipes

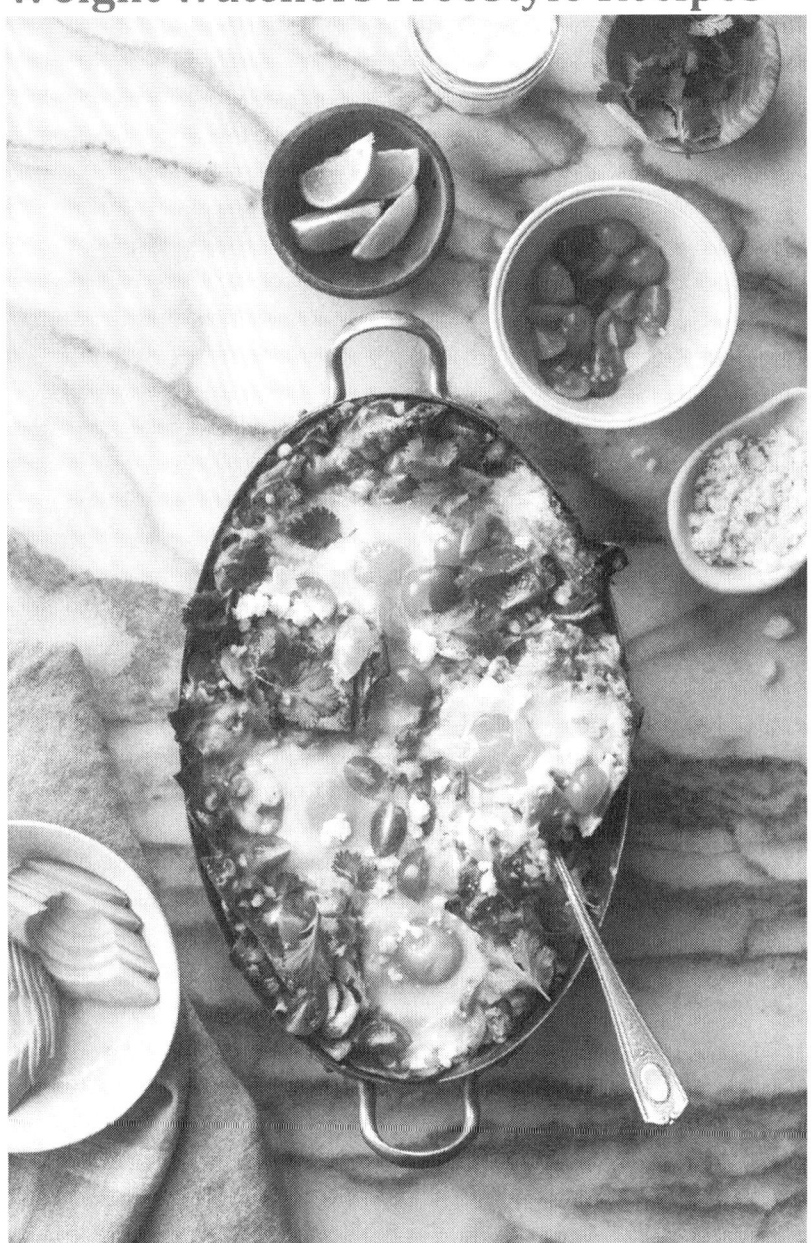

Oregano Balsamic Chicken Lettuce Wraps

Freestyle SmartPoints: 1

Makes 12 servings

Ingredients

- 2 T. lemon juice
- ¼ c. balsamic vinegar
- 2 T. red wine vinegar
- 1 T. honey
- 2 T. water
- 1 t. dried oregano
- ½ t. onion powder
- ½ t. garlic powder
- 1 lb. boneless, skinless chicken breasts
- 1 medium zucchini
- 1 medium red bell pepper
- ½ c. diced red onion
- 8 grape tomatoes
- ½ c. chickpeas
- ½ c. feta cheese
- 1 large head iceberg lettuce
- ⅓ c. plain nonfat Greek yogurt, optional
- Fresh parsley

Instructions

In a small bowl mix the lemon juice, balsamic vinegar, red wine vinegar, honey, water, oregano, onion powder, and garlic powder. In a large sauté pan coated with cooking spray cook the chicken over medium-high heat until it begins to turn white on the outside (about 2 minutes) and add ½ of the vinaigrette to the pan.

Continue to cook until the chicken is cooked through (about 5 additional minutes) and the vinaigrette has evaporated. Remove the pan from the heat and pour the chicken in to a large bowl.

If you prefer the zucchini, bell peppers, and red onions to be cooked, add them to the sauté pan and cook for 2 to 4 minute, or until zucchini becomes soft and the onions become translucent.

In a medium bowl combine the zucchini, bell peppers, onions, tomatoes, chickpeas, and feta with the remaining vinaigrette and stir to combine.

Add the toppings to the cooked chicken and stir to combine. Add the toppings to the cooked chicken and stir to combine. Toss salad with yogurt and parsley just before serving if desired.

To make the lettuce wraps, cut off the stem of the lettuce head and cut in half lengthwise. Peel off individual leaves and wash and pat dry.

Scoop ½ cup of the mixture in each lettuce wrap and top with a dollop of yogurt and fresh parsley if desired.

Mushroom Ginger Chicken Soup

Serves: 5, Serving size: 1 cup, Freestyle SmartPoints: 0

Ingredients
- 1 pound boneless, skinless chicken breast
- 8 ounces fresh mushrooms
- 2 tablespoons lemon juice
- 1 teaspoon garlic, minced
- 1 teaspoon fresh ginger, ground
- 2 cups fat-free chicken broth
- 2 tablespoons reduced-sodium soy
- 3 scallions, thinly sliced
- 1 leek

Instructions

Cook the chicken, mushrooms, lemon juice, garlic and ginger in a medium saucepan over medium heat about 5 minutes.

You may recognize this next step (the leek) from our Creamy Chicken and Stuffing Casserole. (I hope we can all agree that leeks are cool at this point, and totally worth including in this healthy soup).

Meanwhile, cut the top of the leek off (the darkest green part). You will not be using the top half so that part can be discarded.

Slice into the bottom portion of the leek going lengthwise starting about 1-2 inches from the bottom of the leek.

Rotate the leek and slice it the lengthwise again. Do this a couple of more times until you have very thin sliced strips

Now chop the leek into small pieces starting from the top. Rinse the small pieces of the leek.

Add broth, soy sauce, scallions and leek and cook for 7-8 more minutes.

Nutrition Information

Calories: 169, Fat: 3 g, Saturated fat: 1 g, Trans fat: 0 g
Carbs: 3 g, Sugar: 0 g, Sodium: 490 mg, Fiber: 1 g
Protein: 22 g, Cholesterol: 68 mg

Delicious Slow Cooker Chicken

Freestyle SmartPoints: 0

Ingredients:
- 8 chicken breast
- 3/4 teaspoon kosher salt
- freshly ground black pepper
- cooking spray
- 5 garlic cloves, finely chopped
- 1/2 large onion, chopped
- 1 28-ounce can crushed tomatoes
- 1/2 medium red bell pepper, chopped
- 1/2 medium green bell pepper, chopped
- 4 ounce sliced shiitake mushrooms
- 1 sprig of fresh thyme
- 1 sprig of fresh oregano
- 1 bay leaf
- 1 tablespoon chopped fresh parsley
- 1 grated Parmesan cheese, for serving (optional)

Instructions:

   Season the chicken with salt and pepper to taste. Heat a large nonstick skillet over medium-high heat. Coat with cooking spray, add the chicken, and cook until browned- 2 to 3 minutes per side. Transfer to your slow cooker.

   Reduce the heat under the skillet to medium and coat with more cooking spray. Add the garlic and onion and cook, stirring, until soft- 3 to 4 minutes. Transfer to the slow cooker and add the tomatoes, bell peppers, mushrooms, thyme, oregano and bay leaf. Stir to combine.

   Cover and cook on high for 4 hours or on low for 8 hours.

Discard the bay leaf and transfer the chicken to a large plate. Pull the chicken meat from the bones shred the meat, and return it to the sauce. Stir in the parsley. If desired, serve topped with Parmesan cheese.

Nutritional information:
Calories: 220, Fat: 6g, Sat Fat: 1.5g, Cholesterol: 123mg, Sodium: 319mg, Carbohydrates: 10g, Fiber: 2g, Sugar: 6g, Protein: 31g

Yummy Vegetarian Chili

Makes 8: 1 cup/servings

Freestyle SmartPoints: 1

Ingredients:

- 2 cans (15 oz. each) kidney beans
- 1 can (8 oz.) tomato sauce
- 1 can (14.5 oz.) diced tomatoes
- 1 packet (1 oz.) chili seasoning mix
- 1 pkg. (13.5 oz.) Garden Beefless Ground

Instructions:

Mix kidney beans, tomato sauce, diced tomatoes, and chili seasoning in a large stockpot. Allow to cook on medium heat for 5-7 minutes.

Add the beefless ground and cook an additional 5 minutes, or until heated through.

Top with whatever you like.

Nutrition Information:

Serving size: 1 cup, Calories: 153, Fat: 2 g

Saturated fat: 0 g, Unsaturated fat: 0 g, Trans fat: 0 g

Carbohydrates: 20 g, Sugar: 4 g, Sodium: 561 mg

Fiber: 7 g, Protein: 14 g, Cholesterol: 0 mg

Tasty Grilled Shrimp Kebabs

Serve: 8, Serving Size: 1 kebab, Freestyle SmartPoints: 0

Ingredients:
- 32 jumbo raw shrimp, peeled and deveined3 cloves garlic, crushed
- 24 slices (about 3) large limes, very thinly sliced into rounds (optional)
- olive oil cooking spray
- 1 tsp kosher salt
- 1 1/2 tsp ground cumin
- 1/4 cup chopped fresh cilantro, divided
- 16 bamboo skewers soaked in water 1 hour
- 1 lime cut into 8 wedges

Instructions:
Heat the grill on medium heat and spray the grates with oil.

Season the shrimp with garlic, cumin, salt and half of the cilantro in a medium bowl.

Beginning and ending with shrimp, thread the shrimp and folded lime slices onto 8 pairs of parallel skewers to make 8 kebabs total.

Grill the shrimp, turning occasionally, until shrimp is opaque throughout, about 1 to 2 minutes on each side.

Top with remaining cilantro and fresh squeezed lime juice before serving.

Nutrition Information
Calories: 74, Total Fat: 1g, Saturated Fat: g, Chol: 94mg
Sodium: 384mg, Carbohydrates: 3g, Fiber: 1g
Sugar: 0g, Protein: 13g

Delicious Lime Asparagus Chicken

Serve: 4, Serving Size: 1.5 cups, Freestyle SmartPoints: 2

Ingredients:
- 1.33 lbs. boneless skinless chicken breast tenderloins
- 2 tbsp. almond flour
- 1 tsp. garlic powder
- 1/2 tsp. pepper
- 1/2 tsp. salt
- 1 lemon (juiced)
- 1 tbsp. olive oil
- 2 cups asparagus, chopped
- 2 cloves garlic, minced
- 1/2 cup low sodium chicken broth
- 1 tbsp. white wine vinegar

Instructions:

Combine the flour, garlic powder, lemon, salt, and pepper. Toss the chicken with this until all the pieces are just coated.

Heat the olive over medium high heat. Add the chicken and cook on each side for 2-3 minutes until browned. Remove and set aside.

Add the asparagus and garlic to the skillet and cook for 2-3 minutes, stirring often

Add the chicken broth and vinegar to the skillet. Stir and scrape any browned bits off the bottom of the pan. Add the chicken and let simmer for 5-10 minutes on low heat or until chicken is fully cooked. Squeeze the rest lemon juice over top.

Nutritional Information:

Calories 239, Total Fat 5g, Saturated Fat 1g

Cholesterol 0mg, Dietary Fiber 2g, Sugars 2g

Protein 38g

Yummy Chicken Skewers

Serving: 4, Freestyle SmartPoints: 1

Ingredients:
- ¼ cup low sodium soy sauce
- 2 oz. canned pineapple juice
- ¼ cup light coconut milk
- 2 tablespoons honey
- 2 garlic cloves, minced
- 1 tablespoon grated ginger
- ½ teaspoon sesame oil
- 2 scallions, chopped
- 1 lb. fresh pineapple, cut into bite-sized pieces
- 1 ½ pounds (24 oz.) raw boneless, skinless chicken breasts, cut into bite sized chunks
- You'll also need 12" skewers

Instructions:

To create the marinade, combine the soy sauce, pineapple juice, coconut milk, honey, garlic, ginger, sesame oil, and scallions and mix thoroughly.

Pour marinade into a gallon Ziploc bag and add chicken. Seal bag and shake to coat chicken in the marinade. Place the bag in the refrigerator so that the chicken is covered in the marinade and refrigerate for 4 hours.

Pre-heat the grill until hot. Divide the chicken and pineapple evenly onto the eight skewers.

Place the skewers directly on the grill or a skewer rack over the grill over low heat.

Cooking yours for about 5-6 minutes and then flipping them and continuing to cook until chicken is cooked through.

Nutrition Information:

220 calories, 6 g carbs, 4 g fat, 41 g protein, 1 g fiber

Delicious Noodle Chicken Soup

Serve: 10

Serving Size: 1.5 cups

Freestyle SmartPoints: 2

Ingredients:

- 1 lb. boneless, skinless chicken breast
- 1/2 tsp. pepper
- 1 medium onion, chopped
- 1 tbsp. EVOO
- 6 garlic cloves, minced
- 3 celery ribs, sliced
- 3 medium carrots, sliced
- 2 tbsp. dried parsley flakes
- 4 tsp. Italian seasoning
- 12 cups fat-free chicken broth
- 3-1/2 cups uncooked egg noodles

Instructions:

Heat oil in a large stockpot. Sauté onion, celery, and carrots in oil until onion is tender.

Add garlic and cook one minute longer.

Add the chicken broth, chicken, parsley, Italian seasoning. Bring to a boil. Reduce heat; cover and simmer for 20 minutes.

Stir in noodles. Return to a boil and cook 7-9 more minutes, or until the noodles are soft. Add salt and pepper to taste.

Oregano Cumin Chili Chicken

Yield: 8 (1 cup) servings, Freestyle SmartPoints: 1

Ingredients:
- 1 tablespoon Canola oil
- 2 cups yellow onion, chopped
- 2 tablespoons chili powder
- 1 tablespoon minced garlic
- 2 teaspoons ground cumin
- 1 teaspoon oregano
- 3 (15.5 oz.) cans Great Northern beans, rinsed and drained
- 4 cups reduced sodium fat free chicken broth
- 3 cups chopped or shredded cooked skinless chicken breast
- 1 (14.5 oz.) can diced tomatoes
- 1/3 cup chopped fresh cilantro
- 2 tablespoon fresh lime juice
- ½ teaspoon salt
- ½ teaspoon pepper

Instructions:

Bring oil to medium heat in a large pot or Dutch oven. Add the onions and sauté for 5-8 minutes or until tender. Add the chili powder, garlic and cumin and stir to coat the onions.

Cook for 2 more minutes. Add the oregano and beans, stir and cook for 30 more seconds. Add the broth and reduce the heat to medium-low. Simmer for 20 minutes, stirring occasionally.

Remove 2 cups of the bean/broth mixture into a blender and process until smooth. Return pureed mixture to the pot. Add the chicken and tomatoes and cook over medium-low for another 30 minutes, stirring occasionally. Add the cilantro, lime juice, salt & pepper and stir to combine before serving.

Nutrition Information:
291 calories, 36 g carbs, 4 g sugars, 4 g fat, 1 g saturated fat, 27 g protein, 12 g fiber

Delight Marinated Chicken

Serve: 6

Freestyle SmartPoints: 2

Ingredients:

- 2 tablespoons olive oil
- 1 tablespoon red wine vinegar
- 1 tablespoon soy sauce
- 1 tablespoon Worcestershire sauce
- 1 teaspoon ground mustard
- 2 garlic cloves
- Pepper, to taste
- 1-1/2 pounds chicken

Instructions

Mix together the first eight ingredients. Put marinade in a bowl or a Ziploc bag, and add chicken. Refrigerate 4 hours or overnight.

Grill chicken until cooked.

Nutrition Information:
Calories: 158, Fat: 7 g, Saturated fat: 6 g, Fiber: 0 g
Protein: 21 g, Cholesterol: 0 mg

Chili Jalapeno Salsa Roasted Salmon

Serving size: 1 fillet with salsa

Freestyle SmartPoints: 0

Ingredients:

- 1 medium plum tomato, roughly chopped
- 1/2 small onion, roughly chopped
- 1 clove garlic, minced
- 1 small jalapeño pepper, seeded and roughly chopped
- 1 teaspoon cider vinegar
- 1/2 teaspoon chili powder
- 1/4 teaspoon ground cumin
- 1/4 teaspoon salt
- 2 to 3 dashes hot sauce
- Two 4-ounce salmon fillets

Instructions:

Preheat oven to 400°F.

Place tomato, onion, garlic, jalapeño, vinegar, chili powder, cumin, salt and hot sauce in a food processor; process until finely chopped and uniform.

Place salmon in a medium roasting pan; spoon the salsa on top. Roast until the salmon is just cooked through, 12 to 15 minutes.

Nutritional Information

Calories: 211, Fat: 10g, Saturated Fat: 1.75g, Sugar: 1.87g, Fiber: 1.10g, Protein: 25g, Cholesterol: 70.3mg, Carbohydrates: 4.5g

Oregano Celery Turkey Chili

Freestyle SmartPoints: 1, Serves: 8

Ingredients
- 2 cups shredded cooked turkey
- ½ cup diced onion
- ½ green pepper, diced
- ½ cup diced celery
- 2 tablespoons olive oil
- 1 tablespoon minced garlic
- 2 cups chicken broth
- 3 cans (15-16 oz.) white beans
- ¼ teaspoon cayenne pepper
- 1 teaspoon ground cumin
- ¾ teaspoon oregano
- ½ teaspoon salt
- ¼ teaspoon ground black pepper
- shredded Parmesan cheese, sour cream, and cilantro for serving if desired

Instructions:

In a large stock pot or Dutch oven, add onion, green pepper, celery and olive oil. Cook on medium-high heat until onions are translucent and peppers are tender. Stir in garlic.

Add chicken broth, beans, and turkey and mix well. Stir in seasonings. Heat to boiling then reduce heat to simmer and cover for 30-60 minutes, stirring occasionally.

Heat to boiling then reduce heat to simmer and cover for 30-60 minutes, stirring occasionally.

Serve with sour cream, cheese, and cilantro.

Nutritional Information Calories: 460, Fat: 5.6g, Saturated Fat: 1.1g, Sugar: 2.5g, Fiber: 19g, Cholesterol: 64mg,

Delicious Caramelized Garlic Pork Chops

Serve: 6, Free Style Smartpoints: 3

Ingredients

- ½ lbs. Lean pork chops, fat removed
- 2-3 Tbsp. Soy sauce
- 1-2 tsp. Paprika
- 1 large or 2 small onions
- Cooking spray

Instructions

Preheat the grill pan be sure to trim off the fat from the pork chops, if there is any.

Sprinkle the pork chops with paprika.

Spray the grill pan with cooking spray. Set pork chops on the grill. Pour soy sauce over the pork.

Flip the pork chops over. Cover the chops with the grill press, if you have one. Cook five minutes.

While pork chops are cooking, slice onions. I slice mine kind of thick.

Flip the pork chops over again and allow to cook for another five minutes. Once fully cooked, transfer pork chops to a plate.

Cook onion on the grill pan for about 5 minutes, or until slightly softened and caramelized. The onions will pick up the flavor from the pork chops.

Serve and enjoy

Yummy Grilled Chicken Nuggets

Serve: 8, Free Style Smartpoint: 2

Ingredients:
- 2 lbs. boneless skinless chicken
- ½ cup ketchup
- ⅓ cup brewed coffee
- ¼ cup packed brown sugar
- ⅛ cup apple-cider vinegar
- 1 garlic clove, minced
- ½ tsp. salt
- ⅛ tsp. red pepper flakes

Instructions

Spray grill pan with nonstick spray. Preheat grill to medium or medium-high heat.

Cut chicken into small pieces.

Combine ketchup, coffee, brown sugar, vinegar, garlic, ¼ tsp. salt, and pepper flakes in medium saucepan and set over medium heat. Cook, stirring, until mixture comes to a boil.

Reduce heat and simmer 10 minutes.

Meanwhile, Sprinkle chicken with remaining ¼ teaspoon salt. Place chicken on grill pan and allow to cook, turning occasionally, 10-15 minutes.

Brush chicken with sauce, and grill until instant-read thermometer inserted in center registers 165 degrees and the sauce begins to caramelize on the chicken, about 5-10 minutes longer.

Nutrition Information:
Calories: 234, Fat: 4 g, Saturated fat: 0 g, Sugar: 7 g
Sodium: 243 mg, Fiber: 0 g, Protein: 24 g, Chol: 92 mg

Buffalo Chicken in A Slow Cooker

Yield: 12 (1/2 cup) servings

Freestyle SmartPoints: 1

Ingredients:

- 3 lbs. raw boneless skinless chicken breasts
- 12 oz. bottle of Buffalo wing sauce
- 1 oz. packet of dry Ranch mix
- 2 tablespoons light butter

Instructions

Place the chicken breasts in your slow cooker. Pour the bottle of wing sauce over the top of the chicken. Sprinkle the packet of ranch mix over the top of the wing sauce. Place the lid on your slow cooker. Cook on low for 7-9 hours until meat shreds easily.

Remove meat and shred it using two forks. Return shredded meat to the sauce and add the butter. Stir to combine. Continue to cook on low for another hour so the meat can soak up the sauce. Serve however you like!

Nutrition Information:

175 calories, 1 g carbs, 0 g sugars, 5 g fat, 1 g saturated fat, 28 g protein, 0 g fiber

Simple Salad Egg Sandwiches

Serve: 5 Sandwiches

Free Style Smartpoints: 3

Ingredients:

- 6 hard-boiled eggs
- 2 tablespoons tarter sauce
- 1 tablespoon mustard
- 1 teaspoon sugar
- 10 slices light bread

Instructions

Chop up the hard-boiled eggs.

Mix tarter sauce, mustard, and sugar into the eggs.

Scoop ¼ cup egg salad mixture onto 5 pieces of bread and top each with another piece of bread. Cut sandwiches in half.

Nutrition Information:

Calories: 169

Fat: 8 g

Saturated fat: 0 g

Sugar: 3 g

Sodium: 344 mg

Fiber: 4 g

Protein: 13 g

Cholesterol: 198 mg

Tasty Pork Ragu

Serve: 10

Free Style Smarpoint: 1

Ingredients:

- 18 oz. pork tenderloin
- 1 teaspoon kosher salt
- black pepper, to taste
- 1 tsp olive oil
- 5 cloves garlic, smashed with the side of a knife
- 1 (28 oz. can) crushed tomatoes
- 1 small jar roasted red peppers, drained
- 2 sprigs fresh thyme
- 2 bay leaves
- 1 tbsp. chopped fresh parsley, divided

Instructions:

Season pork with salt and pepper. Heat a large pot or Dutch oven over medium-high heat, add oil and garlic and sauté until golden brown, 1 to 1 1/2 minutes;

Remove with a slotted spoon. Add pork and brown about 2 minutes on each side. Add the remaining ingredients to the pot including the garlic, reserving half of the parsley.

Bring to a boil, cook covered on low until the pork is tender, and shreds easily, about 2 hours. Remove bay leaves, shred the pork with 2 forks and top with remaining parsley. Serve over your favorite pasta.

Nutrition Information:

Calories: 93, Total Fat: 1.5g, Saturated Fat: g

Carbs: 6.5g, Fiber: 0g, Sugar: 3g, Protein: 11g

Tasty Tenderly Chicken Baked

Serve: 4

Free Style Smartpoints: 2

Ingredients:

- 4 teaspoons flour
- ½ teaspoon paprika
- 1.25 lbs. raw boneless skinless chicken breast tenderloins
- 2 egg whites, beaten
- ½ cup cornflake crumbs
- ½ teaspoon dried parsley flakes
- ½ teaspoon salt
- ¼ teaspoon black pepper
- ¼ teaspoon cayenne pepper
- ¼ teaspoon onion powder
- ¼ teaspoon garlic powder

Instructions:

Pre-heat the oven to 375 degrees. Line a baking sheet with parchment paper and set aside.

In a small dish, mix together the flour and paprika. Place the chicken strips into a gallon Ziploc bag and add the flour/paprika mixture. Seal the bag and shake to coat the chicken.

In a shallow dish, beat the egg whites and set aside. In a separate shallow dish, stir together the cornflake crumbs, parsley, salt, pepper, cayenne, onion powder and garlic powder.

One at a time, take the flour-coated chicken strips and coat them in the egg whites and then press them into the dish of corn flake crumbs and flip so that both sides are coated in crumbs. Transfer the crumb-coated strips to the prepared baking sheet.

When all the chicken tenders are coated and on the baking sheet, spray the tops of them with cooking spray and place in the oven to bake for 18-20 minutes until cooked through.

Nutrition Information:

229 calories, 12 g carbs, 1 g sugar, 4 g fat, 1 g saturated fat, 35 g protein, 0 g fiber

Sunday Mouth-Watering Steak

Serve: 4

Free Style Smartpoints: 3

Ingredients

1-1/2 teaspoons fresh basil, chopped

1-1/2 teaspoons fresh parsley, chopped

2 teaspoons minced garlic

½ teaspoon salt

¼ teaspoon black pepper

1 pound lean steak

Instructions

Mix the first 5 ingredients together.

Coat the tops and bottoms of the steak with the garlic/seasoning mixture.

Grill 4 minutes on each side or until desired

Nutrition Information:

Calories: 183, Fat: 9 g, Saturated fat: 4 g, Sugar: 0 g
Fiber: 0 g, Protein: 24 g, Cholesterol: 75 mg

Basil Sausage Cannellini Beans Soup

Serve: 4

Free Style Smartpoint: 3

Ingredients

- 10 oz. sweet turkey Italian sausage
- Cooking spray
- 1 onion
- 4 garlic garlic cloves
- 1 (15 oz.) can cannellini beans
- 1 (14.5 oz.) can stewed tomatoes
- 1 (14 oz.) can fat-free less sodium chicken broth
- 2 c. baby spinach
- 1 T. chopped fresh basil
- 2 t. chopped fresh oregano
- 2 T. grated Parmesan cheese

Instructions

Remove casings from sausage. Cook sausage in a large saucepan coated with cooking spray over high heat until browned, stirring to crumble.

Add onion and garlic to pan; cook 2 minutes. Stir in ½ cup water, beans, tomatoes, and broth. Cover and bring to a boil. Uncover and cook 3 minutes or until slightly thick. Remove from heat, and stir in spinach, basil, and oregano. Spinach will begin to shrink in the soup. Ladle 1-1/2 cups soup in each of 4 bowls, and sprinkle each serving with 1-1/2 tsp. Parmesan cheese.

Nutrition Information:

Calories: 272, Fat: 9 g, Saturated fat: 2 g, Sugar: 8 g
Sodium: 1268 mg, Fiber: 9 g, Protein: 21 g

Chapter 3 Conclusion

Thank you again for purchasing my book!

I hope you've enjoyed this book, and if you don't mind, would you please leave an honest review for this book on Amazon? It'd be greatly appreciated!

Thank you and good luck!

Book Number 2

WEIGHT WATCHERS

By Anthony Young

The Ultimate Smart Points Recipes Cookbook, Lose Fat The Smart Way With Weight Watchers

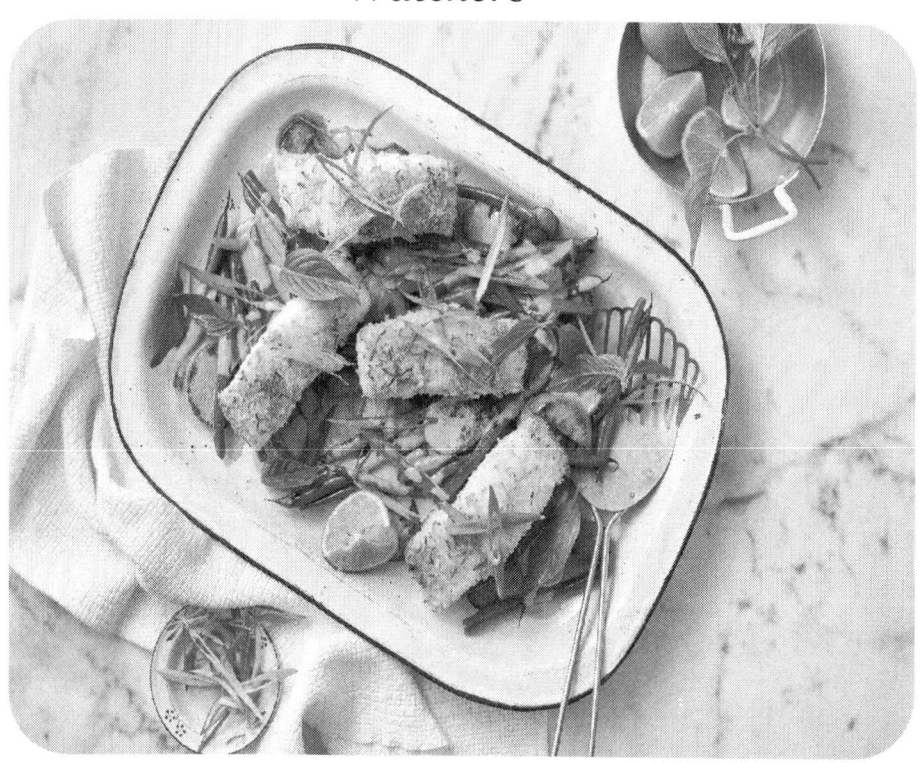

Introduction

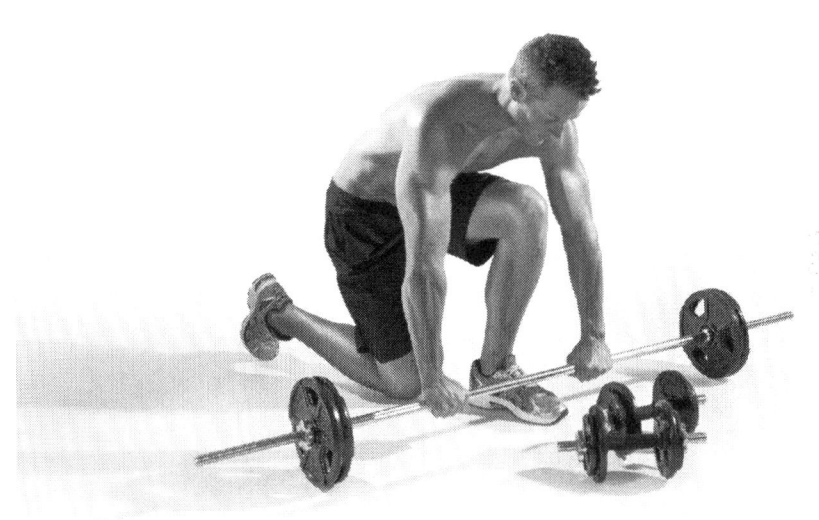

I want to thank you and congratulate you for purchased the book, *"Weight Watchers: The Ultimate Smart Points Recipes Cookbook, Lose Fat The Smart Way With Weight Watchers"*.
This book contains proven steps and strategies on how to lose weight, stay lean for life and live happy.

The Weight Watchers program has been so popular for a number of years now, and it is one of the ultimate, proven, successful ways for people to lose weight. The Weight Watchers plans are so easy for you to follow. It is a program that helps people to stay leaner, thinner but stronger, it's the healthier diet plan.

The human mind and body respond best when they feel safe and relaxed. If you tell someone to get out of their comfort zone the wrong way, then they will respond by rejecting the
Whole idea of change.

While you're on a diet plan, it should be relaxing and enjoyable. You'll want to give your body the greatest gift of all: "GREAT HEALTH & HAPPINESS"

By applying this Weights Watchers program plan, you will find that the fat not only melts away, it stays away. You'll be fitter and happier than you have ever been before, because you'll be adopting the same kind of positive mindset that keeps men and women like you at a healthy weight.

Chapter 1: What is Weight Watchers?

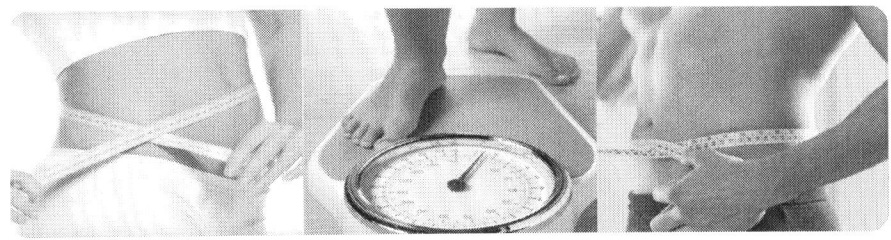

First off, let's have a look at what exactly Weight Watchers is so that you get a firm understanding of it.

The Weight Watchers program is a derivative of the American company of the same name, Weight Watchers International. Founded in the year 1963, it has now spread out to operate in almost 30 different countries apart from the US, and with great success. Their programs have helped many people lose weight using a scientific approach and they also produce and sell various products and packages to help them in this endeavor. Their program is well researched and has stunning results with a healthy and effective approach. This program has worked very well for a majority of the people who have tried it. No wonder it has gained such renown.

So let's begin. First off, you need to sign up for Weight Watchers. You may choose from three different plans, all based on the Weight Watchers program. There's the 'Online Only 'plan, 'Online with Meetings 'plan or even the 'Online with Coaching 'plan. There is a small starter fee for when you first join up, and any other expenses will depend on the plan you've chosen and the period of time you want to be using the package.

Weight Watchers also has various offers you can claim to reduce the overall cost of the program. Joining their online community is also another source of support, and checking out their website and magazine is always a big help with inspiring stories of how others have gained success in weight loss using this program.
These can be massive forms of help and motivation to you, especially to newcomers and those lacking motivation.

Weight Watchers programs are often based on a point system that orders each food by a numbered value, and you may only eat up until you reach a certain point value.

What makes this diet so great is that it does not restrict yourself from eating the foods you love from your diet. It's simply a matter of keeping count of the points according to the food you eat in that day, and not eating any more after you've passed the limit. In this way, the overall plan makes you more health conscious and encourages you towards making better food choices for your health in the long term.

You may still eat all the foods that you love, but since you're watching your weight via a point system, it should help you understand that some of these foods are not great for your body. By limiting the consumption of such foods, you'll do your body much more good in the end.

We will explain specifically how Weight Watchers and its point system works further along in the book. You can also search up on the internet about what Weight Watchers customers think after they have seen all the positive effects of being on the Weight Watchers dieting program.

In fact, looking up a list of best diets, you will find that Weight Watchers is among the top rated ones, just like it has been for a long time now. The diet is well researched and ranked at the top for being healthy and effective compared to most others.

Since the Weight Watchers diet is tracked using a **point-based system**, it is no longer necessary to keep track of calories like so many other diet require you to do. You need to keep track of the points according to the Weight Watchers food points system. It is not unlike a budget, in that you can only spend a particular number of points in a day. The point limit is not fixed, and decided based upon the individual themselves. So you'll be eating what you love, but within a limit.

In doing so, they will teach you about the foods that are good for you and your body, and how much of these foods you will need for your body to be at its healthiest and best condition.

By following the diet, it will teach you about food quantities and the timing of eating as well. The Weight Watchers dieting program will help you make health conscious choices in your day-to-day life. This is precisely what helps you lose weight effectively.

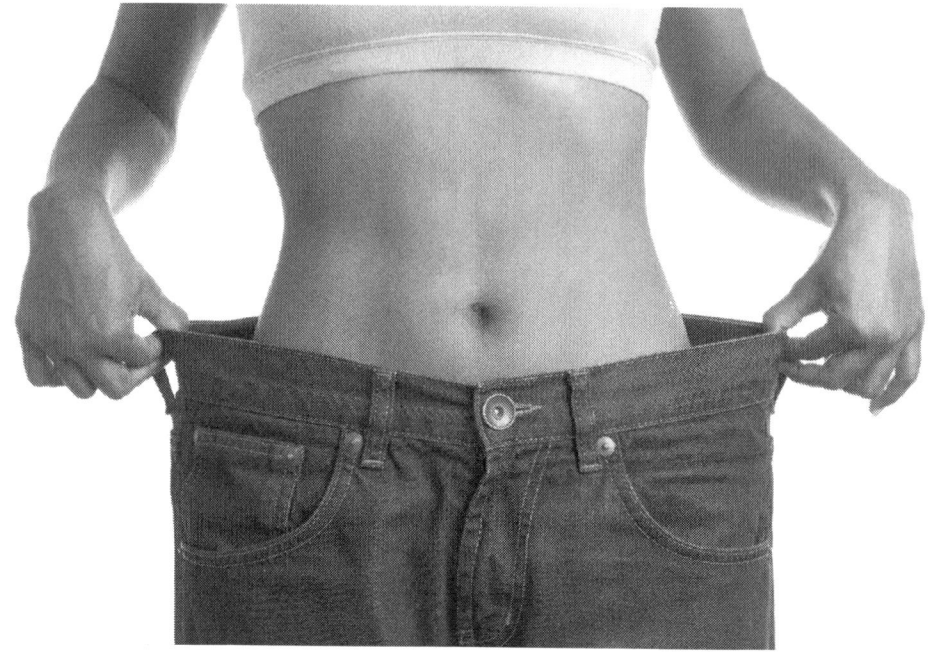

The Various Weight Watchers Plans

Let us have a look at the various Plans available at Weight Watchers:

As we've mentioned before, you may choose from three different types of plans when you sign up for Weight Watchers. You may choose a plan according to what suits your needs and is a possible goal for you as well. The first option is 'OnlinePlus', second is Meetings along with 'OnlinePlus' and thirdly is Coaching with 'OnlinePlus'. The cost rate for each of the plans are estimated per week, and per the plan itself. However, again, there are offers that come up from time to time that you can grab in order to save a bit of money.

- OnlinePlus lets you register and follow the plan structure online at any time. Being online, it can cover all aspects of your diet whenever and wherever. You also get support 24/7 and can access it from anywhere digitally. The OnlinePlus program is what most people start off with since it is the most flexible out of the three. There are many tools that the program uses to make it easy for the customer to follow the program online. The online community forum boards is also a great place to get guidance and support from fellow Weight Watchers.

- Meetings in addition to the OnlinePlus program can be even more beneficial than OnlinePlus alone. You'll meet others who are also following the same system and understand it better. You'll get all the same OnlinePlus tools to access whenever you need just as with the first plan, but the extra support and guidance that the meetings will give you will help you go a long way, especially in staying positive, as you might struggle to lose weight in the early stages of the plan. These meetings are a highly recommended part of what Weight Watchers offers, and since they have a great range of locations for meet-ups, it is easy to attend as well.

- The Coaching option is for those who want individual support at all times. Obviously, you'll get the OnlinePlus access just the same as the last two plans. However, in addition to this, you'll get a coach you'll tailor a specific plan that works for you. The coaches in the program take into account the individual's lifestyle, habits and daily schedule. Using this knowledge, they formulate a plan that enables you to go about your daily living without interfering with a healthy weight loss process.

You may contact them at any time, through calling or texting in case you are in need of some support or advice. Other than that, the tools available to you online should be more than enough to help you keep on track while losing weight.

You can choose any one of these three plans to get you started on your Weight Watchers journey, and once you begin seeing results, you will know exactly why so many people have been vouching for this program for many years.

What does it mean by 'Points'?

What sets Weight Watchers apart from other diets is the fact that it uses a point system to monitor your diet.

The points are a unique feature you're going to love when it comes to starting on this diet plan. The points will tell you the quantity of food that you have left when it comes to eating that day and staying within your general calorie allotment–even though you don't count calories on this diet.

The point system focuses more on the specific macro and micro nutrients of the foods you're eating rather than the calories, which in turn gives you a better outlook on how your body is obtaining its nutrient resources.
A huge majority of diet plans will spend their time and focus looking at the calories of the foods that you eat.

While it is true that eating less calories will help you lose weight, what's even more important is it also matters what type of calories you are eating. For example, eating ten cookies a day may be within your calorie count for that day, but there is no nutrition in them, and all that sugar that you take in an s a result will be hard on your health in the long term.

Foods that have a larger number of good micro and macronutrients are denoted by a lower point value in the Weight Watchers scheme.

Foods that have a high sugars and saturated fat content are going to get a higher point value. You can choose to eat these options if you like, but must be very careful if you don't want to use up all your points without getting the nutrition that you would need for the day. That would end up with you feeling hungry and dissatisfied, and harshly impact upon your weight loss outlook.

If you've chosen to partake in meetings, when you go to your first meeting, your team leader will sit down and talk with you to talk about what your goals may be and what you want to achieve in following the program.

This meeting will help you get personalized information for how that weight loss will happen and ensure you that you are starting out with the correct amount of points. Getting the points right is crucial in helping you lose weight, but at the same time, not having so few points that you aren't getting the nutrition that you need every day.

What's good about Smart Points

There are a many benefits that come from using the Smart Point system for your weight loss goals, and this is partly why the Weight Watchers system is so unique and well-loved. Some of the benefits of using this system are as follows:

•The Smart Points will help you select healthier foods that are good for you and your body. You will be docked any time that you choose foods that are high in saturated fats and sugars while those who chose healthier options would be set.

•The Smart Points system got rid of the unhealthy idea that if you exercise more, you can eat more. Most people will overestimate their level of activity, and so this led to them having problems with losing weight. What's more, they were still eating unhealthy foods in the process. With Smart Points, there's no option to add more points if you exercise more, so you can separate the activity that you do from the foods you take in.

• Smart Points are going to put more focus on having a healthier lifestyle. While weight loss is a part of this process, you'll have to understand that building up healthy habits leading towards a healthy lifestyle is much more conducive to this fact than counting calories alone.

The Cons of Smart Points

While there are large number of positives that stems from the points system of the Weight Watchers program, there are some people who have been concerned over the new Smart Points system, especially those who have gotten used to the old Weight Watchers system. Some of the complaints that have come up in regards to these points are as follows:

• There are some people who have worries that this new system makes it a bit harder to select foods because of the lack of flexibility in point/food allocation. Especially if you were used to the old Points Plus system, this change may be difficult for you to adapt to.

• Some of the restrictions imposed are a little harsher than the old system. The point restrictions for eating things like cake and cookies on the new Smart Points program high enough that many people will want to just give up on the whole program altogether.

While it is a big adjustment, if you're serious enough about losing weight, many will not see an issue with these restrictions and will stay on the plan for the betterment of their health.

Once you sign up to Weight Watchers, depending on the plan you've chosen, you will be able to work with a coach, you may go in person to meetings as well as working online.

The coach will be able to fill out your individual profile and figure out your current weight, how much weight you want to lose, your height, age, and other factors that influences your health, which will determine how much weight you can feasibly lose while on the system. Things, like being an older age or the need to lose more weight, will really slow down a person's metabolism and must be taken into consideration.

Given this information, your coach is able to figure out what amount of points is a good starting place for you individually. They will also give you suggestions on how to stay healthy and how to make the right choices for your meals each and every day. Over time, you will be able to meet with your coach throughout the course of the plan and they will adjust the values based on if you need to lose more weight, reduce the amount of weight lost, or to maintain the weight loss that you have already achieved.

Either way, the points value system in Weight Watchers is a great way to get started on the system and will ensure that you are selecting the best foods for you in order to keep healthy, obtain more energy, and lose weight in the process of doing this.

Keep in mind that when you get started on the Weight Watchers diet plan, most of the time, you'll achieve some weight loss, but the process is focusing more on changing the unhealthy parts of your lifestyle choices rather than losing the weight.

There are a large number of dieting programs that will not work using this points system. In essence, they are just going to tell you the foods that you can eat and the ones that you can't. They'll tell you how many calories that you ought to have and will place a huge number of restrictions on you that it is almost too hard to keep up with during day-to-day life. Contrary to this, when you're using the Smart Points system, you don't have so many limitations.

You'll have the freedom to choose those foods all on your own. You won't be stuck with just a few meals that fit in with the diet plan, as a wide variety and combination of foods are good for you.

Once you're ready to try out something new that is going to help you to lose some weight while still allowing you to live your life without ruining your day, Weight Watchers is the greatest option for you.

SmartPoints Values List:

There is a table below you can use to calculate Weight Watchers point values of the foods you eat. It's an important tool that you can use to keep on top of the points you're accumulating each day. If you're looking for something that isn't on the list but you have the nutritional information, you can do a little math and get an idea of the point value. 50 calories = 1 point, 6 grams of fat = 1 point, and you can subtract 1 point for every 4 grams of fiber. So the calculation for something that is 250 calories, 12 grams of fat, and 4 grams of fiber would be: (250/50) + (12/6) - (4/4) = (5) + (2) - (1) = 6 Weight Watchers points."

Beans & Legumes

#	Name	Amount	Points
1	Beans, baked	1/2 cup	5
2	Beans, baked, canned	1/2 cup (4 oz.)	2
3	Beans, baked, deli	1/2 cup (4 oz.)	3
4	Beans, baked, fast food	1 serving	4
5	Beans, baked, vegetarian, canned	1/2 cup (4 oz.)	2
6	Beans, Black, and rice mix (prepared according to package directions)	1 cup	4
7	Beans, Black, cooked	1/2 cup	2
8	Beans, Black, refried	1/2 cup	1
9	Beans, Black, refried, canned, low-fat or fat-free	1/2 cup	1
10	Beans, Black, uncooked	1 pound	31
11	Beans, Cannellini, cooked	1/2 cup	1

#	Name	Amount	Points
12	Beans, Garbanzo, cooked	1/2 cup	2
13	Beans, Garbanzo, uncooked	1 pound	35
14	Beans, Green, cooked	1 cup	0
15	Beans, Kidney, cooked	1/2 cup	1
16	Beans, Kidney, uncooked	1 pound	30
17	Beans, Lima, cooked	1/2 cup	1
18	Beans, Lima, uncooked	1 pound	30

#	Name	Amount	Points
19	Beans, Navy, cooked	1/2 cup	2
20	Beans, Navy, uncooked	1 pound	30
21	Beans, Pinto, cooked	1/2 cup	2
22	Beans, Pinto, uncooked	1 pound	30
23	Beans, Red, and rice	1 cup	5
24	Beans, Red, and rice mix (prepared according to package directions)	1 cup	5
25	Beans, Refried,	1/2 cup	3
26	Beans, Refried, canned	1/2 cup	2
27	Beans, Refried, fat-free, canncd	1/2 cup	2
28	Beans, Refried, with sausage, canned	1/2 cup	5
29	Beans, Wax, cooked	1 cup	0
30	Beans, White, cooked	1/2 cup	2

#	Name	Amount	Points
31	Beans, White, uncooked	1 pound	30
32	Chickpeas, dry	1/3 cup or 2 oz. cooked or 3/4 oz. uncooked	1
33	Daiquiri	1 (3 fl. oz.)	3
34	Daiquiri mix	1/2 cup (4 fl. oz.) mix	3

#	Name	Amount	Points
35	Lentils, dry	1/3 cup or 2 oz. cooked or 3/4 oz. uncooked	1
36	Soybeans, dry	1/3 cup or 2 oz. cooked or 3/4 oz. uncooked	1
37	Sprouts, alfalfa	1 cup (1 oz.)	0
38	Sprouts, bean	1 cup (4 oz.)	0

Beverages (non-alcohol)

#	Name	Amount	Points
1	Apple Cider	1/2 cup (4 fl. oz.)	1
2	Apple Juice	1/2 cup (4 fl. oz.)	1
3	Beer, non-alcoholic	1 can or bottle (12 fl. oz.)	1
4	Coffee mix, flavored, sugar-free (prepared according to package directions)	1 cup (8 fl. oz.) prepared	1

#	Name	Amount	Points

#	Name	Amount	Points
5	Coffee mix, flavored, with sugar (prepared according to package directions)	1 cup (8 fl. oz.) prepared	1
6	Cranberry juice cocktail, low-calorie	1 cup (8 fl. oz.)	1
7	Cranberry juice cocktail, regular	1/2 cup (4 fl. oz.)	1
8	Eggnog, reduced-calorie, without liquor	1/2 cup (4 fl. oz.)	3
9	Eggnog, store-bought, without liquor	1/2 cup (4 fl. oz.)	5
10	Eggnog, without liquor	1/2 cup (4 fl. oz.)	4
11	Fruit cocktail, unsweetened, canned	1 cup (9 oz.)	2
12	Fruit drink mix, powdered	8 fl. oz. prepared	2
13	Fruit juice, combined, any type	1/2 cup (4 fl. oz.)	1
14	Grape juice (carbonated or non-carbonated)	1/2 cup (4 fl. oz.)	1
15	Grapefruit juice, any type	1/2 cup (4 fl. oz.)	1
16	Hot chocolate, homemade, with whipped topping	1 cup (8 fl. oz.)	7
17	Hot chocolate, homemade, without whipped topping	1 cup (8 fl. oz.)	6

#	Name	Amount	Points
18	Ice cream soda	1 (12 fl. oz.)	8

#	Name	Amount	Points
19	Irish coffee	1 (6 fl. oz. with 2 tbsp. whipped cream)	4
20	Latte, made with fat-free milk	1 small (8 fl. oz.)	2
21	Latte, made with fat-free milk	1 tall (12 fl. oz.)	2
22	Latte, made with fat-free milk	1 grande (16 fl. oz.)	3
23	Latte, made with low-fat milk	1 small (8 fl. oz.)	3
24	Latte, made with low-fat milk	1 tall (12 fl. oz.)	4
25	Latte, made with low-fat milk	1 grande (16 fl. oz.)	4
26	Latte, made with whole milk	1 small (8 fl. oz.)	3
27	Latte, made with whole milk	1 tall (12 fl. oz.)	5
28	Latte, made with whole milk	1 grande (16 fl. oz.)	6
29	Lemonade	1 cup (8 fl. oz.)	2

Beverages (alcohol)

#	Name	Amount	Points
1	Beer, regular	1 can or bottle (12 fl. oz.)	3
2	Beer, light	1 can or bottle (12 fl. oz.)	2
3	Black Russian	1 (3 fl. oz.)	5
4	Bloody Mary	1 (5 fl. oz.)	2
5	Brandy	1 1/2 fl. oz.	2

#	Name	Amount	Points
6	Brandy Alexander	1 (3 fl. oz.)	8
7	Champagne	1 small glass or 1/2 cup (4 fl. oz.)	2
8	Cognac	1 1/2 fl. oz.	2
9	Eggnog, with liquor	1/2 cup (4 fl. oz.)	4
10	Gin	1 jigger (1 1/2 fl. oz.)	2
11	Gin and tonic	1 (6 fl. oz.)	4
12	Gin gimlet	1 (2 1/2 fl. oz.)	3
13	Liqueurs, any type	1 jigger (1 1/2 fl. oz.)	4
14	Liquor (gin, rum, scotch, tequila, vodka, whiskey)	1 jigger (1 1/2 fl. oz.)	2
15	Tom Collins	1 (6 fl. oz.)	3
16	Vodka	1 jigger (1 1/2 fl. oz.)	2
17	Vodka gimlet	1 (2 1/2 fl. oz.)	3

#	Name	Amount	Points
18	Whiskey	1 jigger (1 1/2 fl. oz.)	2
19	Whiskey sour	1 (3 fl. oz.)	3
20	Wine cooler	1 (8 fl. oz.)	3
21	Wine spritzer	1 (8 fl. oz.)	2
22	Wine, dessert, dry	2 fl. oz.	1
23	Wine, dessert, sweet	2 fl. oz.	2
24	Wine, light	4 fl. oz.	1

| 25 | Wine, regular, dry | 1 small glass or 1/2 cup (4 fl. oz.) | 2 |

Breads & Crackers

#	Name	Amount	Points
1	Animal crackers	13(1 oz.)	3
2	Bagel, any type	1 small or 1/2 large (2 oz.)	3
3	Banana Bread	1 slice (5" x 3/4")	5
4	Banana Bread, with nuts	1 slice (5" x 3/4")	5
5	Boston brown bread	1 slice (3 3/4" x 1/2") or 1 1/2 oz.	2
6	Bread crumbs, dried	3 tbsp (3/4 oz.)	1
7	Bread crumbs, dried	1 cup	9
8	Bread crumbs, seasoned	3 tbsp.	2
9	Bread, any type (white, wheat, rye, Italian, French, pumpernickel)	1 slice (1 oz.)	2
10	Bread, cocktail(party-style), any type	2 slices (3/4 oz.)	1
11	Bread, high-fiber, (3 grams or more dietary fiber per slice)	1 slice (1 oz.)	1
12	Bread, Indian(Navajo)fry	1 (5" diameter)	6
13	Bread, reduced-calorie, any type	2 slices (1 1/2 oz.)	1
14	Breadstick, soft	1 (1 1/4 oz.)	2

#	Name	Amount	Points
15	Breadsticks	2 long (7 1/2" x 1/2") or 4 short (5" x 1/2")	1

#	Name	Amount	Points
16	Croissant, chocolate-filled	1 (5" long) or 1 3/4 oz.	6
17	Croissant, plain	1 (5" long) or 1 3/4 oz.	5
18	Date nut bread	1 slice (5" x 1/2")	5
19	Fadge	1 cup	3
20	Flatbreads	3/4 oz.	1
21	Focaccia	1 piece (10" diameter)	25
22	Focaccia bread, any type, store-bought	2 oz.	3
23	Garlic bread, frozen	1 piece	4
24	Graham cracker crumbs	2 tbsp.	1
25	Graham crackers	2 (2 1/2" squares) or 1/2 oz.	1
26	Graham crackers, chocolate-covered	2 (1/2 oz.)	2
27	Graham crackers, mini, any variety	3/4 oz.	2
28	Hamburger bun,	1	3
29	Hamburger bun, light,	1	2
30	Hamburger bun, reduced-calorie	1	1

#	Name	Amount	Points
31	Irish soda bread	1/12 of 8" round loaf or 3 1/2 oz.	5
32	Lavash	1/4 of 10" cracker or 2 1/4 oz.	6

Cereal

#	Name	Amount	Points
1	Cereal, Cold, any type (other than those listed below)	1 cup	2
2	Cereal, Cold, Bran Flakes	3/4 cup	1
3	Cereal, Cold, fortified	1 cup	2
4	Cereal, Cold, frosted	1 cup	3
5	Cereal, Cold, granola	1/2 cup	4
6	Cereal, Cold, granola, homemade	1/2 cup	6
7	Cereal, Cold, granola, low-fat	1/2 cup	3
8	Cereal, Cold, nuggets	1/2 cup	3
9	Cereal, Cold, puffed	1 cup	1
10	Cereal, Cold, raisin bran	3/4 cup	1
11	Cereal, Cold, shredded wheat	1 biscuit	1
12	Cereal, Cold, whole-grain	1 cup	2
13	Cereal, Hot, cream of rice	1 cup	2

#	Name	Amount	Points
14	Cereal, Hot, cream of wheat	1 cup	2
15	Cereal, Hot, farina, cooked	1 cup	2
16	Cereal, Hot, farina, uncooked	1/4 cup	3
17	Cereal, Hot, grits	1 cup	3
18	Cereal, Hot, grits, uncooked	1/4 cup	3
19	Cereal, Hot, oatmeal, cooked	1 cup	3

#	Name	Amount	Points
20	Cereal, Hot, oatmeal, flavored, cooked	1 packet	3
21	Cereal, Hot, oatmeal, uncooked	1 cup	6
22	Hominy grits	1 cup cooked (9 oz.) or 1 1/2 oz. uncooked	2
23	Hominy, whole	1 cup cooked	2
24	Kasha (buckwheat groats)	1 cup cooked or 2 oz. uncooked	3
25	Millet	1/3 cup cooked or 3/4 oz. uncooked	1
26	Quinoa	2 tbsp. dry (3/4 oz.)	1
27	Wheat germ	3 tbsp. (3/4 oz.)	1
28	Wheat germ	1 tsp.	0

Cheese

#	Name	Amount	Points
1	Cheese ball, store-bought	2 tbsp. (1 oz.)	3
2	Cheese, cheddar, soup, canned(made with low-fat or skim milk)	1 cup	4
3	Cheese, cheddar, soup, canned(made with whole milk)	1 cup	5
4	Cheese, cottage, 1% or nonfat, with fruit	1/3 cup	2
5	Cheese, cottage, 1%, 2%, or nonfat	1/3 cup (2 3/4 oz.)	1
6	Cheese, cottage, regular or 4%	1/3 (2 1/2 oz.)	2
7	Cheese, low-fat, hard or semisoft	1 slice, 1 (1") cube, 3 tbsp. shredded, 2 tbsp. grated or 3/4 oz.	2
8	Cheese, Neufchatel	1 tbsp. (1/2 oz.)	1
9	Cheese, nonfat, hard or semisoft	1 slice, 1 (1") cube, 3 tbsp. shredded, 2 tbsp. grated, or 3/4 oz.	1
10	Cheese, pot	1/3 cup	1

#	Name	Amount	Points

#	Name	Amount	Points
11	Cheese, regular, hard or semisoft	1 slice, 1 (1") cube, 3 tbsp. shredded, 2 tbsp. grated, or 3/4 oz.	2
12	Cheese, ricotta, nonfat	1/3 cup	1
13	Cheese, ricotta, part-skim	1/3 cup	3
14	Cheese, ricotta, whole milk	1/3 cup	4
15	Fromage frais (soft cheese with fruit)	3 1/2 oz.	3
16	Soy cheese, nonfat	1 slice, 1 (1") cube, 3 tbsp. shredded, 2 tbsp.grated or 3/4 oz.	1
17	Soy cheese, regular	1 slice, 1 (1") cube, 3 tbsp. shredded, 2 tbsp. grated or 3/4 oz.	2

Condiments, Dressings, Marinades & Spreads

#	Name	Amount	Points
1	Arrowroot	1 tsp.	0
2	Bacon bits, imitation	1 tsp	0
3	Baking powder or soda	1 tsp.	0
4	Bean dip, fat-free	1/2 cup (4 oz.)	1
5	Beets, pickled	1/2 cup	1
6	Chutney	1 tbsp.	1
7	Cocktail sauce	1/4 cup	1

#	Name	Amount	Points
8	Concentrated yeast extract	1 tsp.	0
9	Cream, clotted (English double devon cream)	2 tbsp.	4
10	Cream, light (coffee/table cream)	2 tbsp (1fl. oz.)	2
11	Cream, medium	2 tbsp. (1 fl. oz.)	2
12	Cream, whipped, homemade (no sugar added)	1/4 cup	3
13	Cream, whipping, heavy or light	2 tbsp. (1 fl. oz.)	3
14	Dip, any type	2 tbsp.	2
15	Dip, Artichoke, baked	1/4 cup	6
16	Dip, Spinach	1/4 cup	5
17	Eggs, substitute, fat-free	1/4 cup	1
18	Etouffee mix	2 tbsp. mix	1

#	Name	Amount	Points
19	Filo dough, frozen	1 oz. (about 1 1/2 sheets)	2
20	Fructose	1 tbsp	1
21	Giardeniera (vegetable medley, without olives, packed in vinegar)	1 cup	0
22	Guacamole	1/4 cup	2
23	Guacamole, store-bought	1/4 cup (2 oz.)	2

#	Name	Amount	Points
24	Gumbo base (seasoning mix)	1 1/2 tbsp. (1/2 oz.)	1
25	Hazelnut and chocolate spread	1 tbsp. (1/2 oz.)	2
26	Herring, pickled	1/2 cup	2
27	Honey	1 tbsp.	1
28	Honey	1 cup	20
29	Hummus, any type	1/4 cup	3
30	Hummus, store-bought	1/4 cup	2
31	Hush puppy mix	1/4 cup mix (1 oz.)	3
32	Ketchup	1/4 cup	1
33	Phyllo dough, frozen	1 oz. (about 1 1/2 sheets)	2
34	Sweet and sour mix	1/2 cup (4 fl. oz.) mix	2

Dairy Products

#	Name	Amount	Points
1	Buttermilk baking mix	3 tbsp.	2
2	Buttermilk, dry	1/4 cup powder	2
3	Buttermilk, nonfat, 1%, 1.5%, or 2%	1 cup (8 fl. oz.)	2
4	Cream cheese, light or whipped	2 tbsp. (1 oz.)	1
5	Cream cheese, nonfat	4 tbsp. (2 oz.)	1
6	Cream cheese, regular	1 tbsp. (1/2 oz.)	1
7	Cream cheese, tofu	2 tbsp. (1 oz.)	2
8	Creamer, nondairy	2 tbsp liquid (1 fl. oz.)	1

#	Name	Amount	Points
9	Creamer, nondairy	1 tbsp. powder	1
10	Creamer, nonfat, flavored	2 tbsp. liquid (1 fl. oz.)	1
11	Dairy shake, reduced-calorie	1 packet	2
12	Yogurt and cucumber salad	1/4 cup	1
13	Yogurt bar, chocolate-covered	1	5
14	Yogurt drink	1 cup (8 fl. oz.)	5
15	Yogurt, low-fat, sweetened with sugar, flavored(vanilla, lemon, coffee)	1 cup	4
16	Yogurt, low-fat, sweetened with sugar, fruit-flavored	1 cup	5

#	Name	Amount	Points
17	Yogurt, plain	1 cup	4
18	Yogurt-covered pretzels	7 (8 oz.)	3
19	Yogurt-covered raisins	2 z.	3

Desserts & Sweet Treats

#	Name	Amount	Points
1	Ambrosia	1/2 cup	2
2	Angel Food Cake	1/16 of 10" tube or 2 oz.	2
3	Apple Brown Betty	1 cup	5

#	Name	Amount	Points
4	Apple crisp	3/4 cup	8
5	Apple, baked	1 large	7
6	Apple, candied	1 large	10
7	Apple, caramel	1 large	9
8	Apple, dried	1/4 cup (3/4 oz.)	1
9	Baba au rhum	1	8
10	Bakalava, store-bought	1 piece (1 1/2 oz.)	5

#	Name	Amount	Points
11	Baked Alaska	1 piece (2" wedge)	5
12	Baklava	1 piece (2" square)	5
13	Banana Split	1 serving (3 scoops ice cream, 1 banana, 3 tbsp. syrup, and 1/2 cup whipped cream)	19
14	Bananas Foster	1 serving (2 scoops ice cream, 1/2 banana and 1/3 cup sauce)	16
15	Beef Wellington	1 slice (3 1/2" x 2 1/2" x 1 1/2") or 5 oz.	12
16	Beignet	1 (2" diameter)	2
17	Beignet, from mix (prepared according to pkg. directions)	1	3

#	Name	Amount	Points
18	Brioche	1 (1 oz.)	3
19	Brownie	1 (2" square)	5
20	Brownie, fat-free, store-bought	1 (1 1/2 oz.)	2
21	Brownie, low-fat, store-bought	1 (1 1/2 oz.)	3
22	Cake mix, light, without icing	1/12 of prepared 9" cake	4
23	Cake, cupcake, creme-filled, store-bought	1	4
24	Cake, fat-free, store-bought	1 slice (3 1/2 oz.)	4
25	Cake, snack, creme-filled, store-bought	2 (2 1/4 oz.)	6
26	Cake, sugar-free, store-bought	1 slice (2 1/2 oz.)	5
27	Cake, with icing	1/12 of 9" layer cake or 3" square	12
28	Cake, with icing, store-bought	1 slice (3 oz.)	7
29	Candy corn	1 oz.	2
30	Candy, Caramels	1 oz.	2
31	Candy, Chocolate, any type	1 oz. (2 assorted pieces, 1/2 candy bar, or 2 tbsp. chips)	4
32	Candy, Gumdrops	1 oz.	2
33	Candy, Hard	1 oz.	2
34	Candy, Jellybeans	10 (1 oz.)	2

| 35 | Candy, Licorice | 1 rope (43" long) | 1 |

Fats & Oils

#	Name	Amount	Points
1	Bacon fat	1 tbsp.	3
2	Brewer's yeast	1 tsp.	0
3	Creme fraiche	2 tbsp.	3
4	Lard	1 tbsp.	3
5	Oil, vegetable	1 tsp.	1
6	Oil, vegetable	1 cup	58
7	Textured vegetable protein	1/3 cup (3/4 oz. dry)	1
8	Vegetable oil	1 tsp.	1
9	Vegetable shortening	1 tsp.	1

Fish

#	Name	Amount	Points
1	Anchovies	6(3/4) or 1 tsp. paste	1
2	Bass, striped, coooked	1 fillet (6 oz.)	4
3	Bluefish, cooked	1 fillet (6 oz.)	4
4	Boullabaisse, any type	2 cups	7
5	Carp, cooked	1 fillet (6 oz.)	7
6	Catfish, cooked	1 fillet (6 oz.)	4
7	Cod, cooked	1 fillet (6 oz.)	4
8	Crayfish, canned	1/2 cup or 4 oz.	2
9	Crayfish, cooked	1/2 cup (2 oz.)	1
10	Fish amandine	1 fillett (6 oz.)	13

#	Name	Amount	Points
11	Fish, Anchovies, canned in oil, drained	6	1
12	Fish, Baked, stuffed	1 serving	8
13	Fish, Bass, striped, cooked	1 fillet (6 oz.)	5
14	Fish, Blackened	1 fillet (6 oz.)	12
15	Fish, Bluefish, cooked	1 fillet (6 oz.)	6
16	Fish, Carp, cooked	1 fillet (6 oz.)	7
17	Fish, Catfish, cooked	1 fillet (6 oz.)	6
18	Fish, Cod, cooked	1 fillet (6 oz.)	4
19	Fish, Dried	1 oz.	2

#	Name	Amount	Points
20	Fish, Eel	1 oz.	2
21	Fish, Flounder	1 fillet (6 oz.)	4
22	Fish, Fried	1 fillet (6 oz.)	12
23	Fish, Grouper	1 fillet (6 oz.)	4
24	Fish, Haddock, cooked	1 fillet (6 oz.)	4
25	Fish, Halibut, cooked	1 fillet (6 oz.)	5
26	Fish, Herring, cooked	1 oz.	1
27	Fish, Mackeral, canned	1/2 cup	3
28	Fish, Mackeral, cooked	1 fillet (6 oz.)	8
29	Fish, Mahimahi(dolphinfish), cooked	1 fillet (6 oz.)	4
30	Fish, Perch, cooked	6 oz.	4
31	Fish, Pike, cooked	1 fillet (6 oz.)	4
32	Fish, Pollock, cooked	6 oz.	4
33	Fish, Pompano, cooked	6 oz.	9

#	Name	Amount	Points
34	Fish, Rockfish, cooked	1 fillet (6 oz.)	4
35	Fish, Salmon, canned	1/2 cup (4 oz.)	4
36	Fish, Salmon, cooked	1 fillet (6 oz.)	7
37	Fish, Salmon, grilled, frozen	3 oz.	2
38	Fish, Salmon, smoked	1 oz.	1

#	Name	Amount	Points
39	Fish, Sardines, canned in oil, drained	5	3
40	Fish, Smelt, cooked	1 oz.	1
41	Fish, Snapper, cooked	1 fillet (6 oz.)	4
42	Fish, Sole, cooked	1 fillet (6 oz.)	4
43	Fish, Stuffed, frozen	1 (5 oz.)	5
44	Fish, Swordfish, cooked	1 steak (6 oz.)	4
45	Fish, Trout, cooked	1 fillet (6 oz.)	8
46	Fish, Trout, rainbow, cooked	1 fillet (6 oz.)	6
47	Fish, Tuna, canned in oil, drained	1/2 cup	5
48	Fish, Tuna, canned in water	1/2 cup	3
49	Fish, Tuna, cooked	1 fillet (6 oz.)	6
50	Fish, Tuna, grilled, frozen	1 oz.	2
51	Fish, Whitefish, smoked	2 oz.	1
52	Fish, Whiting, cooked	6 oz.	4
53	Grouper	1 fillet (6 oz.)	4

#	Name	Amount	Points
54	Haddock	1 fillet (6 oz.)	4
55	Halibut	1 fillet (6 oz.)	4
56	Herring fillets, store-bought	1/4 cup (2 oz.)	3

#	Name	Amount	Points
57	Herring, chopped	1/4 cup	4
58	Herring, cooked	1 oz.	2
59	Shark, cooked	1 steak (6 oz.)	4
60	Smelt, cooked	1 oz.	1
61	Sole, cooked	1 fillet (6 oz.)	4
62	Swordfish, cooked	1 steak (6 oz.)	4
63	Trout, rainbow, cooked	1 fillet (6 oz.)	4
64	Tuna dinner in a box (prepred according to package directions)	1 cup prepared	7
65	Tuna, canned in oil, drained	1/2 cup (4 oz.)	5
66	Tuna, canned in water, drained	1/2 cup (4 oz.)	3
67	Tuna, cooked	1 steak (6 oz.)	4
68	Tuna, grilled, frozen	3 oz.	2
69	Tuna-noodle casserole	1 cup	14
70	Whitefish and pike, large, store-bought	1(1 1/4 oz.)	2
71	Whitefish and pike, small, store-bought	2(1 oz.)	2
72	Whitefish salad, store-bought	1 1/2 oz.	5
73	Whiting, cooked	1 fillet (6 oz.)	4

Fruit

#	Name	Amount	Points
1	Apple,fresh	1 large (8 oz.)	2
2	Apple,fresh	1 small (4 oz.)	1
3	Apples, mountain	3 (2"x 1 7/8")	1
4	Apples,crab	2 oz. or 1/2 cup	1
5	Apricots,dried	6 halves (3/4 oz.)	1
6	Apricots,fresh	3 (4 oz.)	1
7	Apricots,unsweetened,canned	1 cup (9oz.)	2
8	Avacado	1/4 (2 oz.)	2
9	Avacado	1/4 (2 oz.)	2
10	Banana	1 medium (6 oz.)	2
11	Blackberries	1 cup (5 oz.)	1
12	Blueberries	1 cup (5 oz.)	1
13	Boysenberries	1 cup (5 oz.)	1
14	Breadfruit,uncooked	1 cup (8 oz.)	4
15	Cantaloupe	1/4 melon (8 oz.) or 1 cup (5 oz.)	1
16	Carambola (star fruit)	1 (5 oz.)	1
17	Casaba melon	1 cup (6 oz.)	1
18	Cherries,dried	1/4 cup (1 1/2 oz.)	2

#	Name	Amount	Points
19	Cherries,fresh	1 cup (5 1/2 oz.)	1

#	Name	Amount	Points
20	Coconut,cream of	1/4 cup (2 fl. oz.)	5
21	Coconut,shredded	1 tsp.	0
22	Currants,dried	1/4 cup (1 1/2 oz.)	2
23	Currants,fresh	1 cup (4 oz.)	1
24	Fig,dried	1 (3/4 oz.)	1
25	Fig,fresh	1 (2 oz.)	0
26	Fruit,candied	2 tbsp.	1
27	Fruit,dried,mixed	1/4 cup (1 1/2 oz.)	2
28	Fruit,spreadable	1 1/2 tbsp.	1
29	Gooseberries	1 cup (5 oz.)	1
30	Grapefruit	1 (16 oz.)	2
31	Grapefruit sections	1 cup (9 oz.)	1
32	Grapes	1 cup, 20 small or 12 large	1
33	Green papaya	1 cup	1
34	Guava	1 (4 oz.) or 1/3 pulp	1
35	Honeydew melon	1/8 (6 oz.) or 1 cup	1
36	Jackfruit	1/2 cup	2
37	Kiwi fruit	1 (4 oz.)	1

Grains & Rices

#	Name	Amount	Points

#	Name	Amount	Points
1	Barley	1 cup cooked or 1/4 cup uncooked	3
2	Bran, Corn, uncooked	1/4 cup	0
3	Bran, Oat, uncooked	1/4 cup	1
4	Bran, Rice, uncooked	1/4 cup	2
5	Bran, Wheat, uncooked	1 tbsp.	0
6	Bran, Wheat, uncooked	1/4 cup	0
7	Bulgur, uncooked	1/4 cup	2
8	Corn dog	1 (2 3/4 oz.)	5
9	Corn on the cob	1 small ear (5") or 4 oz.	1
10	Corn, baby (ears)	1 cup	1
11	Corn, kernels or cream-style	1 cup (6 oz.)	2
12	Cornstarch	1 tsp.	1
13	Flour, any type	1 tsp.	0
14	Flour, any type	3 tbsp. (3/4 oz.)	1
15	Flour, Potato	1 tsp.	0
16	Flour, Potato	1/4 cup	2
17	Flour, White	1 cup	9
18	Flour, White	3 tbsp.	1
19	Flour, White	1 tsp.	0
20	Flour, Whole Wheat	1 cup	8
21	Flour, Whole Wheat	3 tbsp.	1
22	Flour, Whole Wheat	1 tsp.	0

#	Name	Amount	Points
23	Rice (crisp) and marshmallow treat	1 small (3/4 oz.)	2
24	Rice dirty	1 cup	9
25	Rice mix, flavored, any type	1/2 cup prepared	3
26	Rice, dirty, mix (prepared without fat)	1 cup prepared	3
27	Rice, fried, chicken or pork, frozen	1 cup	2
28	Rice, fried, with beef, chicken, pork, or shrimp	1/2 cup	8
29	Rice, Spanish	1 cup	5
30	Rice, Spanish, canned	1 cup (9 oz.)	3
31	Rice, white	1 cup	4
32	Rice, wild	1 cup cooked	3
33	Seeds, caraway	1 tsp.	0
34	Seeds, poppy	1 tsp.	0
35	Seeds, pumpkin or sunflower	1 tbsp.	1
36	Seeds, sesame	1 tsp.	0

Meats

#	Name	Amount	Points
1	Antelope, cooked	1 oz.	1
2	Armadillo, cooked	1 oz.	1
3	Bacon, Canadian-style	1 slice (1 oz.)	1
4	Bacon, cooked, crisp	3 slices	3
5	Bacon, reduced-fat, cooked, crisp	3 slices	3

#	Name	Amount	Points
6	Bacon, turkey, cooked, crisp	3 slices	2
7	Bear, black, cooked	1 oz.	2
8	Beaver, cooked	1 oz.	1
9	Beef and Broccoli	1 cup	4
10	Beef and broccoli, frozen	1 cup (7 oz.)	5
11	Beef Bourguignon	1 1/2 cups	18
12	Beef jerky or stick	1 oz.	3
13	Beef, Bourguignon	1 1/2 cups	20
14	Beef, corned, canned	1 slice (2 oz.)	3
15	Beef, dried, store-bought	7 slices (1 oz.)	1
16	Beef, Ground, country-fried, store-bought	1 patty (4 oz.)	8
17	Beef, Ground, lean, cooked	1 patty (3 oz.)	6
18	Beef, Ground, lean, cooked	1/2 cup (2 oz.)	4

#	Name	Amount	Points
19	Beef, Ground, lean, cooked(round or loin cuts with all visible fat trimmed)	1 slice or 1/2 cup cubed or shredded (2 oz.)	3
20	Beef, Ground, lean, uncooked	1 pound	22
21	Beef, Ground, regular, cooked	1 patty (3 oz.)	6
22	Beef, Ground, regular, cooked	1/2 cup (2 oz.)	4

#	Name	Amount	Points
23	Beef, Ground, regular, cooked	1 patty (3 oz.)	6
24	Beef, Ground, regular, uncooked	1 pound	25
25	Beef, Orange-Ginger	1 cup	11
26	Beef, regular, cooked	1 slice or 1/2 cup cubed or shredded (2 oz.)	4
27	Beef, steak, cooked	1 small (4 oz.)	7
28	Beef, steak, cooked	1 small (4 oz.)	7
29	Beef, steak, lean (round or loin cuts with all visible fat trimmed), cooked	1 small (4 oz.)	5
30	Beef, steak, lean (round or loin cuts with all visible fat trimmed), cooked	1 small (4 oz.)	5

#	Name	Amount	Points
31	Beef, Sweet and sour	1 cup	12
32	Beef, Tongue, cooked	1 oz.	2
33	Beefalo, cooked	1 oz.	1
34	Bologna, beef or pork	1 slice (1 oz.)	2
35	Bologna, turkey	1 slice (1 oz.)	1
36	Boudin, store-bought	2 oz.	2
37	Bratwurst	2 oz.	5
38	Buffalo, water cooked	1 oz.	1
39	Caribou, cooked	1 oz.	1
40	Chitterlings	1 oz.	2

#	Name	Amount	Points
41	Chorizo	1 link (5" long) or 3 1/2 oz.	9
42	Crab, deviled	1/2 cup	5
43	Crab, stuffed, frozen	1 (3 oz.)	3
44	Crabmeat, artificial	1/2 cup (3 oz.)	2
45	Crabmeat, canned	1/2 cup or 4 oz.	2
46	Crabmeat, cooked	1/2 cup (2 oz.)	1
47	Duck a l orange	1/4 duck with 2 tsbp. sauce	19
48	Duck with fruit sauce	1/4 duck with skin and 1/2 cup sauce	13

#	Name	Amount	Points
49	Duck, wild or domestic, with skin, cooked	1/4 duck (3 1/2 oz. without bone)	13
50	Duck, wild or domestic, without skin, cooked	1/4 duck (3 1/2 oz. without bone)	5
51	Elk, cooked	1 oz.	1
52	Emu, cooked	1 oz.	1
53	Flanken	2 slices (4 oz.)	8
54	Frankfurter, beef and pork, with cheese	1 (1 3/4 oz.)	5
55	Frankfurter, beef and pork, fat-free	1 (1 3/4 oz.)	1
56	Frankfurter, beef and pork, light	1 (1 3/4 oz.)	2
57	Frankfurter, beef and pork, regular	1 (1 3/4 oz.)	5

58	Frankfurter, chicken	1 (2 oz.)	4
59	Frankfurter, Rolls, light	1 (1 1/2 oz.)	2
60	Frankfurter, Rolls, reduced-calorie	1 (1 1/2 oz.)	1
61	Frankfurter, Rolls, regular	1 (1 1/2 oz.)	3
62	Frankfurter, turkey	1 (2 oz.)	3
63	Frankfurter, turkey, fat-free	1 (1 1/2 oz.)	1

Nuts, Seeds & Butters

#	Name	Amount	Points
1	Almond butter	1 tsp.	1
2	Almonds	22 nuts (1 oz. shelled)	4
3	Brazil nuts	8 nuts (1 oz. shelled)	5
4	Butter, regular	1 cup	51
5	Butter, regular or whipped	1 tsp.	1
6	Cashews, dry-roasted, without salt added	14 nuts (1 oz. shelled)	4
7	Chestnuts	6 small (2 oz.)	1
8	Dates, dried	1/4 cup (5 dates)	2
9	Dates, fresh	2 (3/4 oz.)	1
10	Fruit butter, any type	1 tbsp.	1
11	Hazelnuts	20 nuts (1 oz. shelled)	4
12	Pistachios	40 nuts (1 oz. shelled)	4

| 13 | Soybean nuts | 1/4 cup (1 oz.) | 3 |
| 14 | Walnuts | 14 halves (1 oz. shelled) | 5 |

Pasta

#	Name	Amount	Points
1	Cannelloni, cheese, with meat sauce	2 shells with 1/2 cup sauce	29
2	Cannelloni, cheese, with tomato sauce	2 shells with 1/2 cup a of sauce	14
3	Cannelloni, meat, with cream sauce	2 shells with 1/2 cup sauce	17
4	Cannelloni, meat, with tomato sauce	2 shells with 1/2 cup sauce	14
5	Cannelloni, spinach and cheese, with cream sauce	2 shells with 1/2 cup sauce	15
6	Cannelloni, spinach and cheese, with tomato sauce	2 shells with 1/2 cup sauce	12
7	Cannelloni, with tomato sauce, frozen	7 oz.	6
8	Fettuccini Alfredo	1 cup	16
9	Fettuccini Alfredo, frozen	1 cup (7 oz.)	7
10	Fettuccini with broccoli and chicken in Alfredo sauce, frozen	1 cup (8 oz.)	9
11	Lasagna, cheese, with tomato sauce, frozen	1 package (10 oz.)	8

#	Name	Amount	Points

12	Lasagna, chicken, frozen	1 cup (7 oz.)	5
13	Lasagna, vegetable, frozen	1 cup (7 1/2 oz.)	5
14	Lasagna, vegetable, frozen	1 cup	5
15	Lasagna, vegetarian, with cheese	1 serving	10
16	Lasagna, vegetarian, with cheese and spinach	1 serving	9
17	Lasagna, with meat	1 cup	6
18	Lasagna, with meat sauce, frozen	1 cup (7 1/2 oz.)	6
19	Lasgana noodles, uncooked	2 1/2 or 2 oz.	4
20	Linguine, with red clam sauce	1 cup linguine with 1/2 cup sauce	6
21	Linguine, with white clam sauce	1 cup linguine with 1/2 cup sauce	8
22	Spaghetti with tomato sauce and meatballs	1 cup spaghetti with 1/2 cup sauce	12
23	Tortellini, beef, chicken, or pork, without sauce, frozen	1 cup (3 3/4 oz.)	5
24	Tortellini, cheese, without sauce	10 (2/3 cup)	3
25	Tortellini, cheese, without sauce, frozen	1 cup (3 3/4 oz.)	6

#	Name	Amount	Points
26	Tortellini, meat, without sauce	10 (2/3 cup)	3
27	Tortellini, mushroom, without sauce, frozen	1 cup (3 1/2 oz.)	6
28	Tortellini, sausage, without sauce, frozen	1 cup (3 3/4 oz.)	7

Vegetables

#	Name	Amount	Points
1	Arugula	1 cup	0
2	Asparagus, cooked	1 cup (6 oz.) or 12 spears	0
3	Bamboo shoots	1 cup	0
4	Beets, cooked	1 cup ((6 oz.)	0

#	Name	Amount	Points
5	Bittermelon (balsam-pear pods)	1 cup, cooked	0
6	Bittermelon (balsam-pear pods)	1 cup, uncooked	0
7	Bottle gourd	1 cup	0
8	Broccoli rabe	1 cup	0
9	Broccoli, cooked or uncooked	1 cup or 4 spears	0
10	Brussel sprouts, cooked or uncooked	1 cup (5 oz.)	0
11	Cabbage(all varieties including bok choy, kai choi, won bok, makina, Chinese, swamp, and	1 cup	0

#	Name	Amount	Points
	mustard), cooked or uncooked		
12	Capers	1 tbsp.	0
13	Cardoon	1 cup	0
14	Carob, unsweetened	1 tsp.	0
15	Carrot and raisin salad	1/2 cup	5
16	Carrots and parsnips	1 cup	4
17	Carrots, cooked or uncooked	1 cup	1
18	Cauliflower, cooked or uncooked	1 cup (4 oz.)	0
19	Celeriac (celery root)	1 cup	0

#	Name	Amount	Points
20	Celery	1 cup (2 oz.) or 2 stalks	0
21	Chicory (curly endive)	1 cup or 6 oz.	0
22	Coconut, cream of	1/4 cup (2 fl. oz.)	5
23	Coconut, shredded	1 tsp.	0
24	Cranberries, dried	1/4 cup (1 1/2 oz.)	2
25	Cranberries, fresh	1 cup (4 oz.)	1
26	Cucumber	1 cup, 1 medium, or 4 oz.	0
27	Daikon	1 cup	0
28	Eggplant, cooked	1 cup (3 oz.)	0
29	Endive, Belgain (French)	1 cup (2 oz.)	0
30	Escarole	1 cup	0

31	Fiddlefern (fiddlehead greens)	1 cup	0
32	Gherkins, fresh	1 cup or 1 medium	0
33	Gourd, white, flowered	1 cup	0

Why You Should Attend Meetings:

The Weight Watchers program is benefited hugely from its customers attending and taking part in the meetings organized.
Although it sounds quite overbearing and intimidating, especially for anyone who may be quite self-conscious about their weight? However, I'm sure you will be pleasantly surprised by how these meetings are organized and how they work. You are able to ask others who have attended them as well to get some input. These meetings will help motivate and guide you on your way to reaching your weight loss goal.

There are many other people, just like you, who have been really struggling to lose a certain amount of weight for many years, and may be unhappy with their current weight.

Some people would just be there to get healthier, while others need to lose weight because of health conditions. Whatever the reason, all the members that you will meet have the same overarching goal.

The atmosphere at the meetings organized is friendly and respectful towards everyone present. Since it is also private, you do not have to worry about what you say there.

You are encouraged to introduce yourself and express your experiences once you start attending the meetings. Share something about yourself and talk about what your goal is. These meeting also progressively help the members figure out what works and doesn't work for them, and share their progress in the program. This helps other people with similar problems relate and learn how to get better at managing their health over time. These meetings only take 30-40 minutes and can easily be slotted into your schedule.

You may choose how interactive you want to be at the meeting, and nobody forces you to talk if you don't want to. Start getting comfortable just by listening to other members and you may find that you're becoming more open as well. Having some excess weight and trying to lose it is nothing to be ashamed about, and it's wholly possible for you if you set your mind to it. There are guides at the meeting who are able to help you and share their own success stories whilst on the program. All of this helps you on your journey and also improves your state of mind as well– a crucial part to getting healthy. As we've emphasized before, a healthy mindset is very important and will play a crucial role in achieving your goals.

Why You Should Get A Coach?

You will get advice from proven experts if you chose to partake in the Coaching program. You'll get advice on a one-to-one basis, and these coaches are people who also experienced what you are going through now, and gone way beyond what they have ever imagined. They know exactly what you'll need to do and their advice can help you in sticking with your program as well.

Getting some personalized help in this way can help you go the distance. You have the ability to choose a coach for yourself by looking up their story and expertise levels. The coach you choose will want to know everything there is to know about you and your weight management so far. Tell them about yourself so they understand what your goals are.

Your daily food habits and lifestyle are always accounted for by the coach when he or she makes a specially designed plan that is specifically suited to your life and goals. You will get much more tailored guidance and support compared to the other plans on the program. You can contact them whenever you need through calls, texts or e-mails. This works especially well for people who need a stricter regimen and someone to give them an extra push so that they do not get off track.

Weight Watchers also has a line of products to help members stay healthy and follow the program easily.

They have various packaged foods, exercise equipment, meal prep tools, cookbooks and DVD resources as well. All of these are available for purchase if you so wish, and are designed in a way to let customers go the distance in their weight loss journey.

Oprah Winfrey is an official spokesperson for Weight Watchers and the exposure has helped them gain even more fame. She has tried the program herself and gotten some amazing results like many members that follow the Weight Watchers programs.

So you see, the Weight Watchers program covers a whole host of different aspects of your life. It is a scientifically supported diet program that you follow to lose weight steadily and effectively. It is a program that will help you make the necessary changes in your lifestyle to get to a point where you have instilled in yourself healthy habits for a better lifestyle.

You can learn how to lose weight and build a healthy lifestyle in the simplest way possible. Many people fail to realize that many short-term efforts to lose weight will not show long-term results and lead to a vicious, unsatisfying cycle that will not get you any lasting results. Instead, do it the correct and healthy way. Your body will thank you for it in the end.

DESPERATION TO LOSE weight might bring YOU to start... but knowing YOUR 'WHY' will KEEP YOU GOING

Chapter 2 Weight Watchers Breakfast Recipes

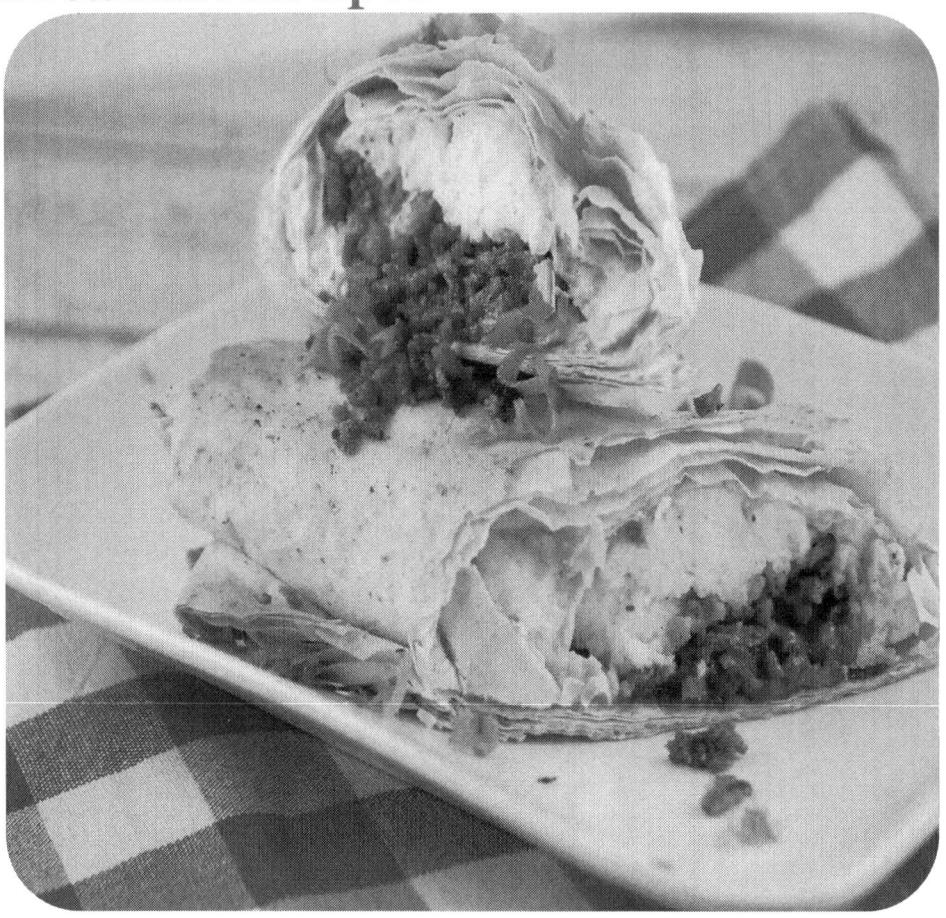

Delicious Asparagus Pancetta Potato Hash

Cooking time: 15
Serves: 2   Smart points: 6
Ingredients:

- 2 large eggs
- 1 ounce pancetta, diced
- 1 medium shallot, chopped
- 8 ounces gold potatoes, peeled, chopped into ½ inch cubes
- ¼ pound asparagus, tough ends trimmed, chopped into ½ inch pieces
- Salt to taste
- Pepper to taste
- Cooking spray

Directions:

1. Place a nonstick skillet or cast iron skillet over medium heat. Spray cooking spray over it.
2. Add pancetta and sauté until golden in color. Remove with a slotted spoon and place on paper towels.
3. Let the fat remain in the pan. Add potatoes and do not stir. Season with salt and pepper. When the underside is brown, stir. Add shallots and sauté until the potatoes are golden brown from all sides. The shallots will also be golden brown by now.
4. Add asparagus and cover the skillet. Cook until the asparagus is tender as well as crisp. Uncover. Taste and adjust the seasoning if necessary. Add the pancetta and stir.
6. Cook the eggs as per your desire. Divide and place hash on individual serving plates. Place the eggs on top and serve.

Calories: 217, Carbohydrate – 22 g, Fiber –4 g, Sugar –1 g, Fat –9 g, Protein – 12 g,

Egg Avocado Toast in a Hole

Cooking time: 20 minutes

Serves: 2

Smart points: 6

Ingredients:

- 2 large eggs
- 2 slices whole wheat or whole grain bread
- Freshly ground black pepper to taste
- Kosher salt to taste
- 2 ounces avocado, mashed
- Hot sauce to taste (optional)
- Olive oil cooking spray

Directions:

1. Make a hole in the center of the bread slices using a cookie cutter of heart shape or slightly bigger round shape. Do not discard the cut part.
2. Add salt and pepper to the avocado.
3. Place a skillet over medium low heat. Spray cooking spray. Place both the bread slices as well as the cut part in the skillet.
4. Break an egg into the hole of the bread. Cook until the egg sets. Sprinkle salt and pepper. Flip sides and cook the other side too. Cook the cut piece too.
5. Remove on to a plate. Top with avocado and hot sauce and serve.
6. Repeat with the 2nd slice of bread.

Calories: 229, Carbohydrate – 23 g Fat – 10 g, Protein – 12 g,

Yummy Lemon Poppy Seeds Muffins

Serves: 12 **SmartPoints: 5**

Ingredients:

- ½ cup sugar
- 2 eggs
- ¼ cup applesauce, unsweetened
- 1 teaspoon vanilla extract
- 1 large lemon, zest and juiced
- ¾ cup plain Greek yogurt (fat free)
- ½ cup white rice flour
- ½ cup oat flour
- ⅓ cup brown rice flour
- 2 teaspoon baking powder
- ½ teaspoon baking soda
- ½ teaspoon salt
- 2 tablespoon poppy seeds
- 2 tablespoon almonds, sliced

Directions:

1. Preheat the oven to 350°F. Either grease a muffin tin lightly, or line it with muffin papers.

2. In a large bowl, cream the following ingredients together: sugar, eggs, applesauce, and vanilla extract. Add the lemon zest to the mixture as well as the lemon juice and Greek yogurt. Mix all the ingredients until they are well combined.

3. Add the white rice flour, oat flour and brown rice flour, baking powder, baking soda, and salt. Mix until the ingredients have been well combined. Put in the poppy seeds and mix them with the other ingredients. Divide the batter among the muffin cups. Sprinkle the almonds on top. Bake for about 20 minutes, or until you insert a toothpick at the center of each muffin, and it comes out clean.

Nutritional Information: Calories 132, Total Fat 3.0 g, Carbohydrate 22.0 g, Protein 5.0 g

Onion Hash Browns Omelet

Serves: 4

SmartPoints: 6

Ingredients:
- 6 slices bacon
- 2 cups hash browns, frozen, or chopped potatoes
- ½ cup onion, chopped
- ½ cup green pepper, chopped
- 4 eggs
- ¼ cup milk
- 1 cup cheese, grated
- Salt and pepper to taste

Directions:

1. Start by cooking the bacon slices in a heavy skillet until they become crispy. Remove them from the pan and set them aside to cool.
2. Mix the hash browns or chopped potatoes, onion and green pepper in the same skillet where you cooked the bacon. The pan will have bacon drippings to cook the mixture.
3. Cook over low heat until the underside of the mixture becomes brown and crispy.
4. Blend the 4 eggs with the milk and then pour this mixture over the potato mixture. Top with the grated cheese and cooked bacon.
5. Cover the skillet with a lid and cook the mixture over low heat for about 20 minutes or until the egg is cooked. Remove from the heat.
6. Cut the omelet into wedges. Sprinkle with salt and pepper to taste. Serve.

Nutritional Information: Calories 514, Total Fat 34.9 g, Total Carbohydrate 30.4 g, Protein 19.0 g

Cheesy Tomato Ham Egg Bake

Serves: 6   **Smart points: 3**

Ingredients:
- 2 large egg whites
- 4 large eggs
- 1 cup low fat cheddar cheese, shredded
- 1 medium tomato, diced
- 2 scallions, sliced
- ¼ cup red bell pepper, chopped
- 2.5 ounces shiitake mushrooms, sliced
- ½ cup broccoli, finely chopped
- 2 teaspoons olive oil
- 3.5 ounces lean ham steak, diced
- 2 tablespoons fat free milk
- Pepper to taste
- Salt to taste
- Cooking spray

Method:

1.   Spray an ovenproof dish with cooking spray. Sprinkle half the cheese in it. Set aside. Place a nonstick skillet over medium heat. Add scallions, mushrooms and red pepper and sauté until tender. Add tomatoes and sauté for a couple of minutes. Add ham and broccoli. Stir and remove from heat. Transfer this mixture over the cheese in the dish. Whisk together in a bowl, eggs, whites, milk, salt and pepper. Pour over the mixture in the dish. Sprinkle the remaining cheese over it. Bake in a preheated oven at 375° F for about 30 minutes or a toothpick when inserted in the center comes out clean. Let it remain in the oven for about 10 minutes. Slice into wedges and serve.

Nutrition Information: Calories: 152, Carbohydrate – 5 g, Fat –8 g, Protein - 14 g

Scallion Eggs Tomato Breakfast

Cooking time: 40 minutes

Serves: 2

Smart points: 3

Ingredients:

- 4 egg whites, whisked
- 1 whole grain English muffin, split
- 2 scallions, minced + extra to scan
- 1 teaspoon olive oil
- ¼ cup low fat Mexican cheese blend, grated
- Black pepper to taste
- Kosher salt to taste
- ¼ cup grape or cherry heirloom tomatoes, quartered

Directions:

1. Toast the muffins in a toaster until the edges are light brown. Alternately, toast it in an oven.
2. Place a skillet over medium heat. Add oil. When the oil is heated, add scallions and sauté until translucent.
3. Add whites, salt and pepper and scramble it. Cook until the eggs are cooked as per your desire.
4. Place over the toasted muffins. Place tomatoes over it followed by scallions and cheese.
5. Broil in a preheated oven for a couple of minutes until the cheese melts.

Nutritional Information: Calories: 160, Carbohydrate – 16 g, Fat –8 g, Protein – 15 g

Cinnamon Pineapple Raisin Bread

Serves: 1

SmartPoints: 4

Ingredients:

- 1 egg (medium)
- ¼ cup canned pineapple (no sugar added), crushed
- ¼ teaspoon cinnamon powder, divided
- 1 slice raisin bread

Directions:

1. Beat the egg in a shallow dish. Add half of the cinnamon and combine.
2. Drain the juice from the pineapple into the egg mixture and beat it again. Prick the slice of bread with a fork on both sides and soak the slice in the egg mixture. Turn the bread many times so it can absorb a lot of egg mixture.
3. Gently transfer the slice of bread to a nonstick baking sheet. Take the drained pineapple and the remaining cinnamon powder and spread it on the bread together with the remaining egg mixture. Bake at 400°F for about 20 minutes, and serve warm.

Nutritional Information:

Nutrition Information: Calories 168, Total Fat 5.6 g, Total Carbohydrate 22.1 g, Protein 7.6 g

Healthy Breakfast Burrito

Serves: 4 **SmartPoints: 5**

Ingredients:

- 2 teaspoons olive oil
- 2 scallions, chopped
- 1 tomato, chopped
- 1 green pepper (or green chili pepper or jalapeno), chopped
- 2 garlic cloves, minced
- 2 large eggs
- 4 egg whites
- 2 tablespoons cilantro, chopped
- ½ cup cheddar cheese (low-fat), chopped
- ¼ teaspoon salt
- ¼ teaspoon pepper
- 4 whole wheat tortillas
- Cooking spray (non-fat)
- ½ cup sour cream (non-fat)
- ½ cup salsa

Directions:

1. Preheat the oven to 400°F. Heat a skillet over medium heat and add the oil. When the oil has heated, add the chopped scallions, tomato, green pepper, and minced garlic. Sauté the mixture for 5 minutes. Add the whole eggs and the egg whites. Cook until the eggs are scrambled, about 3 to 5 minutes. Remove from the heat and add the cilantro, cheese, salt, and pepper as you stir. Spray a baking dish with cooking spray. Place one tortilla on a plate and spoon a quarter of the mixture on top. Roll up the tortilla and place it on the baking dish with the seams facing downwards. Repeat this method with the remaining tortillas. Bake for 10 minutes and then serve with salsa and sour cream.

Nutritional Information: Calories 298, Total Fat 9.3 g, Total Carbohydrate 36.6 g, Protein 17.4 g

Cinnamon Oatmeal Muffin with Applesauce

Serves: 1

SmartPoints: 4

Ingredients:

- 4 teaspoons non-fat milk
- 3 teaspoons wheat bran
- 3 teaspoons whole wheat flour
- 2 teaspoons rolled oats (not instant)
- 2 teaspoons brown sugar
- 2 teaspoons applesauce (unsweetened)
- 2 teaspoons egg beaters
- ¼ teaspoon baking powder
- ¼ teaspoon cinnamon powder
- Cooking spray

Directions:

1. Mix all the ingredients together until just combined. Spray a container (such as a medium-sized ramekin) with nonstick cooking spray. Pour the mixture into the container.
2. Microwave on high for 1 minute or 90 seconds. Allow it to cool, and then serve.

Nutritional Information: Calories 100, Fat 0.5 g, Carbohydrate 20.8 g, Protein 3.2 g

Nutritious Avocado and Pear Smoothie

Serves: 4
SmartPoints: 4

Ingredients:
- 1 Hass avocado, ripe and firm
- 1 cup pear juice, unsweetened
- ½ cup Greek yogurt (nonfat)
- 2 tablespoons honey
- ½ teaspoon vanilla extract
- 2 cups ice cubes

Directions:
1. Cut the avocado in half.
2. Remove the pit and use a spoon to scoop the avocado into a blender.
3. Add the pear juice, yogurt, honey, and vanilla to the blender and puree until the mixture becomes smooth. Add the ice cubes and blend again, and you have a smoothie for your breakfast.
4. Pour the smoothie into 4 glasses and serve.

Nutritional Information: Calories 160, Fat 7.4 g, Carbohydrate 3.4 g, Protein 4.0 g

Artichoke Spinach Breakfast Bake

Serves: 4

Smart points: 4

Ingredients:
- 2 large egg whites
- 4 large eggs
- 5 ounces frozen chopped spinach, thawed, squeezed of excess moisture
- 1/3 cup canned artichokes, drained, pat dried
- ¼ cup scallions, finely chopped
- 1 clove garlic, minced
- 3 tablespoons red bell pepper, chopped
- 2 teaspoons fresh dill, chopped
- 2 tablespoons fat free milk
- ¼ cup feta cheese, crumbled
- 1 tablespoon parmesan cheese, grated
- Salt to taste
- Pepper to taste
- Cooking spray

Directions:

1. Spray a baking dish with cooking spray. Add spinach, scallions, artichoke, red pepper and garlic into it. Mix well and spread all over the dish evenly.
2. Whisk together in a bowl, eggs, whites, milk, salt and pepper. Add Parmesan and feta and stir. Pour over the vegetables in the dish.
3. Bake in a preheated oven at 375° F for about 30 minutes or a toothpick when inserted in the center comes out clean. Slice into wedges and serve.

Nutritional Information: Calories: 128, Carbohydrate – 4 g, Fat –7 g, Protein – 11 g

Hash Browns Bacon & Eggs

Serves: 4   **SmartPoints: 4**

Ingredients:
- 4 hash brown patties, frozen
- 6 egg whites
- 2 large eggs
- 3 ounces Canadian bacon or turkey bacon, finely chopped
- Cooking spray
- 1 tablespoon scallion (the green part), minced
- ⅛ teaspoon black pepper to taste
- ⅛ teaspoon table salt to taste
- **Optional:**
- 8 teaspoons hot and spicy ketchup
- ⅛ teaspoon hot pepper sauce

Directions:

1. Coat a large nonstick skillet with cooking spray. Place the hash brown patties on the skillet and cook over medium heat. Start with one side and cook until they become golden brown, about 7 to 9 minutes. Flip the patties on the other side and cook them until they become golden brown, about 5 minutes.

4. In the meantime, coat another large nonstick skillet with cooking spray and heat it over medium-low heat. Take a large bowl and beat together the 6 egg whites, 2 eggs, chopped Canadian bacon or turkey bacon, minced scallion, the hot pepper sauce (optional), salt, and pepper. Pour the mixture into the skillet and increase the heat to medium. Allow the eggs to set partially and then scramble them using a spatula. When the eggs have set properly, remove the pan from the heat and cover it with a lid until the hash browns have cooked. Place one hash brown patty on each of 4 serving plates. Divide the egg mixture into 4 portions. Top each hash patty with a portion of the egg mixture, and 2 teaspoons of ketchup. Season with salt and pepper if you like, and then serve.

Nutritional Info: Calories 85, Fat 4.0 g, Carbohydrate 0.9 g, Protein 10.6 g

Tasty Basil Zucchini Omelet

Makes: 1 serving

SmartPoints: 4

Ingredients
- ½ teaspoon olive oil
- ½ cup zucchini (diced)
- ½ cup tomatoes (diced)
- 2 tablespoons basil
- 2 eggs
- 1 egg white
- Salt and pepper to taste

Directions:

- Heat oil in a skillet and sauté the tomatoes and zucchini in it, seasoning it with salt and pepper. Mix in the basil and place aside.
- Whisk together the egg white and eggs with some salt and pepper and pour into the pan greased with cooking spray.
- Cook on both sides until done.
- Transfer the egg onto a platter, scoop the sautéed veggies at the centre and then fold the egg over.

Nutritional information :Calories: 205; Total Fat: 12 g; Carbohydrates: 6 g; Proteins: 19 g

Onion Tomato Avocado Scramble

Makes: 4 servings
SmartPoints: 7

Ingredients

- 2 teaspoon olive oil
- 2 cups broccoli (chopped)
- 1 red pepper (chopped)
- ½ cup onion (diced)
- 8 eggs (whisked)
- 1 tomato (diced)
- 1 avocado (chopped)
- Salt and pepper to taste

Directions:

• Heat olive oil in a pan and sauté the onion, broccoli, red pepper in it for 3-4 minutes until crispy tender.

• Mix in the eggs, stirring often until done.

• Mix in the tomato and avocado and season with salt and pepper.

Nutritional information:Calories: 279; Total Fat: 19 g; Carbohydrates: 12 g; Proteins: 16 g

Simple Chia Pudding

Makes: 3 servings
SmartPoints: 6

Ingredients

- 12 cashews
- 3 cups water
- 3 tablespoon hemp seeds
- 3 small dates
- ½ teaspoon cinnamon
- 6 tablespoons chia seeds
- Pinch of sea salt

Directions:

Combine the hemp seeds, dates, cashews and a cup of water in a blender, blending until smooth.

Add in the rest of the ingredients and pulse until mixed.

Refrigerate for 2-3 hours.

Nutritional information:Calories: 236; Total Fat: 15 g; Carbohydrates: 21 g; Proteins: 8 g

Toasted Hazelnuts Apple & Chicken Omelette

Makes: 1 serving

SmartPoints: 12

Ingredients

- 1 teaspoon coconut oil
- 8 egg whites
- 5 ¼ oz. cooked chicken breast (shredded)
- 1 apple (cored, peeled, diced)
- 3 collard leaves (stems discarded, finely chopped)
- ¾ oz. hazelnuts (toasted, crushed)
- Salt and pepper to taste

Directions:

- Heat coconut oil in a skillet and sauté the chicken in it until golden brown.
- Mix in the apple and cook for ½ minute. Transfer onto a platter.
- Add the collards to the skillet and cook for ½ minute.
- Return the chicken mixture back to the skillet and pour the egg whites over.
- Sprinkle the hazelnuts, reduce the flame and cook covered loosely for around 5 minutes.

Nutritional information: Calories: 587; Total Fat: 23.5 g; Carbohydrates: 33.3 g; Proteins: 62.6 g

Oregano Garlic Sweet Potato Spinach Casserole

Makes: 4 servings
SmartPoints: 7

Ingredients

- 2 teaspoon olive oil
- 3 cups sweet potato (peeled, diced)
- ½ red onion (diced)
- ½ teaspoon salt
- ½ teaspoon garlic powder
- ½ teaspoon oregano
- ½ teaspoon pepper
- 4 cups spinach (chopped)
- 8 eggs

Directions:

Heat olive oil in a pan and cook the onion and sweet potatoes in it for 8-10 minutes, adding tablespoons of water to prevent burning.

Season with the spices and add the spinach, cooking until wilted.

Transfer the mixture in a baking dish greased with cooking spray.

Whisk together the eggs and pour it over the veggie mixture.

Bake in an oven preheated to 400 degrees Fahrenheit for 25-30 minutes till the eggs are cooked and set.

Nutritional information: Calories: 264; Total Fat: 12 g; Carbohydrates: 24 g; Proteins: 15 g

Simple Cinnamon Oatmeal Muffin Breakfast

Serves: 1

SmartPoints: 4

Ingredients:

- 4 teaspoons non-fat milk
- 3 teaspoons wheat bran
- 3 teaspoons whole wheat flour
- 2 teaspoons rolled oats (not instant)
- 2 teaspoons brown sugar
- 2 teaspoons applesauce (unsweetened)
- 2 teaspoons egg beaters
- ¼ teaspoon baking powder
- ¼ teaspoon cinnamon powder
- Cooking spray

Directions:

1. Mix all the ingredients together until just combined. Spray a container (such as a medium-sized ramekin) with nonstick cooking spray. Pour the mixture into the container.
2. Microwave on high for 1 minute or 90 seconds. Allow it to cool, and then serve.

Nutritional Information: Calories 100, Total Fat 0.5 g, Carbohydrate 20.8 g, Protein 3.2 g

Basil Garlic Veggie-Egg Breakfast

Makes: 2 servings

SmartPoints: 5

Ingredients

- 1 tablespoon olive oil
- 2 zucchini (chopped)
- 7 oz. cherry tomatoes (halved)
- 1 garlic clove (crushed)
- 2 eggs
- Basil leaves for garnish
- Salt and pepper

Directions:

Heat oil in a pan and sauté the courgettes in it for 5 minutes, stirring often.

Add the garlic and tomatoes and cook for another couple of minutes.

Season with salt and pepper and make two gaps for the eggs.

Crack the eggs into the two gaps and cook covered for 2-3 minutes.

Serve garnished with basil leaves.

Nutritional information : Calories: 196kcal; Total Fat: 13 g; Carbohydrates: 7 g; Proteins: 12 g

Chapter 3 Weight Watchers Main Course Recipes

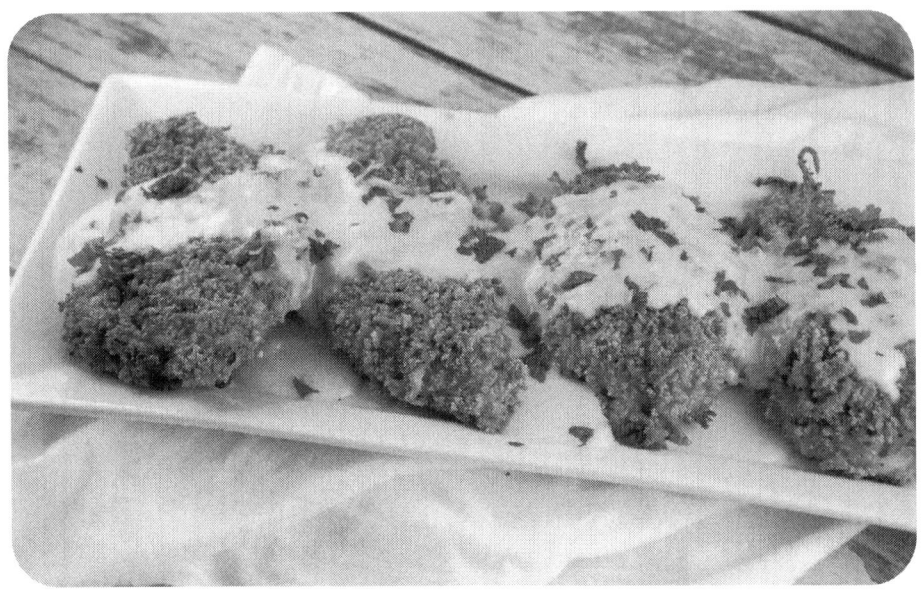

Parsley Garlic Eggplant "Meatballs"

Serves: 12 (4 meatballs each)
Smart points: 6
Ingredients:
- 2 ½ pounds eggplant, unpeeled, cut into 1 inch pieces
- 1 tablespoon olive oil
- 4 cloves garlic, crushed
- 2 large eggs, beaten
- Freshly ground black pepper
- Kosher salt to taste
- 3 cups Italian seasoned breadcrumbs
- 4 ounces Pecorino Romano cheese, freshly grated + extra for serving
- 4 tablespoons fresh basil, chopped + extra to garnish
- 2 tablespoons flat leaf parsley, chopped
- 2 jars (25.25 ounces each) Delallo Pomodoro sauce
- Cooking spray
- Part skim ricotta cheese to serve (optional)

Directions:
1. Take a rimmed baking sheet and spray it with cooking spray. Set aside.
2. Place a nonstick skillet over medium high heat. Add oil. When the oil is heated, add eggplant, salt, pepper, and about ½ cup water. Stir occasionally. Cook until tender. Remove from heat and cool for a few minutes.
3. Transfer into a food processor and pulse for a few seconds until well combined.
4. Transfer into a bowl. Add breadcrumbs, salt, pepper, egg, Romano cheese, garlic, parsley and basil. Mix well.
5. Divide and make 48 balls. Roll it tightly and place on the baking sheet that was set aside. Bake in a preheated oven at 375° F until brown and firm.
7. Pour sauce into a skillet and heat. Add the meatballs into the skillet and simmer for 5-6 minutes. Garnish with basil and top with ricotta if desired.

Nutritional Information: Calories: 222.5, Carbohydrate – 31 g, Fat – 7.5 g, Protein – 10.5 g

Chili Cumin Grilled Steak

Serves 4, **SmartPoints: 9**

Ingredients:
- 3 cups sweet potatoes, cubed
- ½ teaspoon chili powder
- 2 tablespoons rice vinegar
- ¾ cup fresh cilantro, chopped
- ¼ cup low fat sour cream
- 2 cloves garlic, crushed and minced
- 1 teaspoon cumin
- 1 teaspoon lime juice
- 1 pound beef steak, cut into cubes
- 2 cups red bell pepper, chopped into large pieces
- 1 large onion, chopped into large pieces
- 1 tablespoon olive oil, divided
- 1 teaspoon ground black pepper
- ½ teaspoon oregano

Directions
1. Prepare a stovetop grill and preheat the oven to 425°F.
2. On a baking sheet lined with parchment paper, toss together the sweet potatoes, chili powder and enough of the olive oil to lightly coat. Place the baking sheet in the oven and bake while preparing the rest of the ingredients, until the potatoes are firm tender. Remove from the oven and let cool slightly before handling.
3. In a small bowl, combine the rice vinegar, cilantro, sour cream, garlic, cumin, and lime juice. Mix well and set aside.
4. Using wooden or metal skewers, place the steak, sweet potatoes, red bell pepper and onion onto each skewer in an alternating pattern until all ingredients are used.
5. Brush lightly with the remaining vegetable oil, and sprinkle black pepper and oregano.
6. Place the skewers onto the stove top grill and cook, turning once, until steak reaches desired doneness, approximately 5-8 minutes per side.
7. Remove from heat and serve with cilantro sauce.

Nutritional Information: Calories 319, Total Fat 10.9 g, Carbohydrate 30.5 g, Protein 25.9 g

Delicious Beef Stew

Serves 4, **SmartPoints: 7**

Ingredients:
- 1 ½ pounds lean beef stew cut into cubes
- 1 ½ tablespoons flour
- 1 tablespoon black peppercorns
- 1 teaspoon five spice powder
- 4 cloves garlic, crushed and minced
- 1 tablespoon fresh lemongrass, chopped
- 2 tablespoons rice vinegar
- ½ tablespoon low sodium soy sauce
- 1 tablespoon honey
- 2 tablespoons olive oil
- 1 cup red onion, chopped
- 2 cups carrots, chopped
- ½ cup poblano pepper, diced
- 1 tablespoon jalapeno pepper
- 4 cups tomatoes, chopped
- 2 tablespoons tomato paste
- 2 cups acorn squash, cubed
- 3 cups low sodium beef broth
- 1 cinnamon stick
- 2 cardamom pods
- 2 star anise pods

Directions:

1. In a bowl, combine the flour, peppercorns, and five spice powder. Toss the stew meat in the flour mixture, coating generously.
2. Mix in the garlic, lemongrass, rice vinegar, soy sauce, and honey. Mix well and refrigerate for at least 30 minutes.
3. Preheat the oven to 325°F. Add the olive oil to a Dutch oven over medium heat. Add the beef, onions, and carrots. Sauté until meat is lightly browned, approximately 3-5 minutes. Add the poblano and jalapeno peppers, and cook for 1-2 minutes.

6. Add the tomatoes, tomato paste, squash, beef stock, cinnamon stick, cardamom and star anise. Continue to cook, while stirring until well blended, approximately 3-5 minutes.
7. Cover the Dutch oven and place in the oven to bake for approximately 40 minutes, or until the meat is cooked through and tender.

Nutritional Information: Calories 231, Total Fat 7.7 g, Carbohydrate 22.8 g, Protein 19.6 g

Yummy Chili Garlic Thai Chicken

Serves: 4, **SmartPoints: 6**
Ingredients:
- 1 pound chicken breast tenders
- Cooking spray
- ¼ cup garlic chili sauce
- 2 tablespoons honey
- 1 teaspoon salt
- 1 teaspoon black pepper
- 2 cups asparagus spears, chopped
- 1 cup onion, sliced
- 1 tablespoon olive oil
- Cooked rice for serving (optional)

Directions:
1. Preheat the oven to 375°F and spray an 8x8 or larger baking dish with cooking spray.
2. Place the chicken in a single layer in the baking dish and season with the salt and black pepper.
3. In a bowl, combine the garlic chili sauce and honey. Mix well.
4. Pour the sauce mixture over the chicken, using a basting brush to evenly distribute over each piece.
5. Add the asparagus and onion to the baking dish and drizzle with the olive oil.
6. Place the baking dish in the oven and bake for 25-30 minutes, or until the chicken is cooked through.
7. Remove from the oven and let rest for at least 5 minutes before serving.

Nutritional Information: Calories 242, Total Fat 6.6 g, Carbohydrate 17.1 g,, Protein 28.2 g

Delicious Broccoli Pineapple Pork

Serves: 4, **SmartPoints: 8**

Ingredients:
- 1 pound cooked pork, shredded
- 1 tablespoon vegetable oil or cooking spray
- 3 cups broccoli florets
- 1 teaspoon salt
- 1 teaspoon black pepper
- 2 cups medium heat tomato salsa, fresh or jarred
- 2 cups fresh pineapple chunks
- ¼ cup fresh orange juice (or other citrus juice of choice)
- Fresh cilantro for serving (optional)
- Cooked rice for serving (optional)

Directions:

1. Heat the vegetable oil or cooking spray in a large skillet over medium heat.
2. Add the broccoli and sauté for 5-7 minutes, or until crisp tender.
3. Add the shredded pork to the skillet and season with salt and black pepper.
4. Next, add the salsa, pineapple chunks, and orange juice. Mix well.
5. Increase the heat to medium high until the liquid comes to a low boil.
6. Reduce the heat to low, cover, and simmer for 5-7 minutes, or until heated through.
7. Remove from the heat and serve with cooked rice and cilantro, if desired.

Nutritional Information:
Calories 328, Total Fat 10.3 g, Carbohydrate 22.7 g, Protein 37.4 g

Onion Paprika Breaded Veal Cutlets

Serves 4

SmartPoints: 6

Ingredients

- 1 pound veal cutlets, trimmed
- Cooking spray
- 1/2 cup dry whole-wheat breadcrumbs
- 1/2 teaspoon paprika
- 1/2 teaspoon onion powder
- 1/2 teaspoon salt and black pepper
- 4 teaspoons canola oil
- 1 large egg white
- 4 teaspoons cornstarch

Directions

1. Pound the veal cutlet if needed, so they are ½ inch thick.
2. Preheat oven to 400°F. and line a rimmed baking sheet with parchment paper. Spray lightly with cooking spray.
3. Mix breadcrumbs, and spices in a shallow bowl. Add the oil and mix well.
4. Sprinkle cornstarch over the veal cutlets to evenly coat both sides.
5. Beat the egg white until it becomes frothy. Place in a shallow dish.
6. Add the veal cutlets to the egg white. Massage to coat. Add the cutlets one by one to the breadcrumbs and spices mixt. Try to coat as evenly as possible.
7. Arrange the veal cutlets on the baking sheet. Bake in the preheated oven for 15to 18 minutes, until golden and cooked through.

Nutritional Information:

Calories 219, Total Fat 7 g, Carbohydrate 11.2 g, Protein 24.8 g

Asparagus Italian Steak Rolls

Serves: 4, **SmartPoints: 5**

Ingredients:
- 1 pound flank steak, thinly sliced in sheets
- ¼ cup low fat Italian salad dressing
- 1 cup red bell pepper, sliced
- ½ pound asparagus spears, trimmed
- 1 cup onion, sliced
- Cooking spray
- 1 teaspoon salt
- 1 teaspoon black pepper
- Kitchen twine

Directions:
1. Place the steaks in a bowl and cover them with the Italian salad dressing. Toss to coat. Set aside for 15 minutes.
2. Preheat the oven to 350°F and line a baking sheet with aluminum foil.
3. Remove the meat from the marinade and lay the slices out on a flat surface. Season with salt and black pepper as desired.
4. Place the red bell pepper, asparagus and onion pieces on the center of each piece of meat in equal amounts.
5. Roll up each piece of meat around the vegetables and secure with kitchen twine.
6. Heat the cooking spray in a skillet over medium high.
7. Add the steak rolls to the skillet and sear on all sides.
8. Transfer the steak rolls to the baking sheet. Place it in the oven and bake for 15-20 minutes, or until the meat is cooked through and the vegetables are crisp tender.
9. Remove from the oven and let rest 5 minutes before serving.

Nutritional Information:
Calories 211, Total Fat 8.6 g, Carbohydrate 7.9 g, Protein 24.6 g

Garlic Dijon Chicken

Serves: 4

SmartPoints: 3

Ingredients:

- 1 pound boneless, skinless chicken breasts
- 1 tablespoon olive oil or cooking spray
- 1 teaspoon salt
- 1 teaspoon white pepper
- 1 teaspoon fresh thyme
- ¼ cup Dijon mustard
- ½ cup low fat milk
- 2 cloves garlic, crushed and minced
- 4 cups fresh spinach, torn

Directions:

1. Heat the olive oil in a skillet over medium heat.
2. Using a meat mallet, pound the chicken until it reaches a thickness of approximately ¼ inch.
3. Season the chicken with salt, white pepper and fresh thyme. Add the chicken to the skillet and cook for 3-4 minutes per side.
4. Combine the Dijon mustard, milk, and garlic.
5. Add the Dijon mixture to the skillet and cook for 1-2 minutes.
6. Add the spinach and cook an additional 4-5 minutes, turning the chicken occasionally, until the chicken is cooked through and the spinach is wilted.
7. Remove from heat and serve warm with favorite accompaniment.

Nutritional Information:

Calories 170, Total Fat 3.2 g, Carbohydrate 2.6 g, Protein 27.6 g

Onion Leek Red Wine Steak

Serves: 4
SmartPoints: 7
Ingredients:
- 4 lean beef steaks, approximately 4-5 ounces each
- Cooking spray
- 1 teaspoon salt
- 1 teaspoon coarse ground black pepper
- ½ teaspoon onion powder
- ½ teaspoon oregano
- 1 cup leeks, sliced
- ½ cup dry red wine
- 1 cup beef stock
- ¼ cup gorgonzola cheese crumbles

Directions:
1. Heat the cooking spray in a deep skillet over medium-high heat.
2. Season the steaks with salt, black pepper, onion powder and oregano. Place the steaks in the skillet and sear on all sides, then remove and keep warm.
3. Add the leeks to the skillet and sauté for 2-3 minutes.
4. Next, add the red wine and reduce for 2-3 minutes, scraping the bottom of the pan to remove any steak bits.
5. Add the beef stock and return the steaks to the skillet.
6. Bring to a low boil before reducing the heat to medium low and cooking for 7-10 minutes, or until the steaks have reached desired doneness.
7. Remove the skillet from the heat and transfer the steaks to serving plates. Spoon the pan sauce and leeks over the steaks and then garnish with crumbled gorgonzola.
8. Let the steaks rest for 5 minutes before slicing.

Nutritional Information:
Calories 250, Total Fat 10.8 g, Carbohydrate 5.1 g, Protein 26.3 g

Cheddar Broccoli Chicken Noodle Casserole

Serves: 3, **Smart points: 8**

Ingredients:
- 3 ounces Ronzoni Smart taste noodles (or no yolk)
- 2 cloves garlic, thinly sliced
- 2 teaspoons butter
- 1 ½ tablespoons all purpose flour
- ½ cup 1% milk
- 2 ounces reduced fat Sharp cheddar cheese, shredded
- 1 ½ tablespoons parmesan cheese, shredded
- 1 teaspoon oil
- 6 ounces fresh broccoli florets, chopped
- 1 small shallot, minced
- 2/3 cups fat free chicken broth
- 6 ounces cooked shredded chicken breast
- Cooking spray
- 1 tablespoon seasoned bread crumbs

Directions:

1. Cook the noodles according to the instructions on the package until al dente (preferably undercooked)
2. Place a skillet over medium heat. Add oil. When the oil is heated, add garlic and sauté until golden brown. Add broccoli and salt and stir.
3. Cover and cook until the broccoli is slightly tender. Remove from heat and set aside.
4. Spray a small casserole dish with cooking spray and set aside.
5. Place a skillet over medium low heat. Add butter. When the butter melts, add shallots and sauté until translucent. Add flour and salt and stir for a couple of minutes on low heat. Add chicken broth and whisk until well combined. And milk and stir. Stir constantly until it thickens.
6. Remove from heat and add cheddar cheese and half the Parmesan and mix until cheese melts. Add chicken, noodles, and broccoli and mix until well coated.

7. Transfer into the prepared casserole dish. Sprinkle remaining Parmesan and breadcrumbs. Spray a little cooking spray. Bake in a preheated oven at 325° F for about 20 – 25 minutes. Broil for a couple of minutes if your want a brown top.
Nutritional Info: Calories: 313, Carbohydrate – 31.2 g, Fat – 9.9 g, Protein – 27.2 g

Delicious Roasted Leg of Lamb

Serves 8, **SmartPoints: 6**
Ingredients
- 3 bulbs of garlic
- 1 tablespoon lemon zest
- 2 tablespoons fresh thyme, chopped
- 3 teaspoons olive oil, divided
- Teaspoon each of salt and black pepper, or to taste
- 3 ½ pounds boneless leg of lamb, trimmed and tied in a roast

Directions
1. Preheat the oven to 350°F. Line a roasting pan with parchment paper or foil.
2. Mince 4 cloves of garlic from one of the bulbs. Mix in a small bowl the minced garlic, lemon zest, 2 ½ teaspoons of olive oil, thyme, and salt and pepper.
3. Rub the meat with the garlic mixture.
4. Cut the top of the garlic bulbs, about ½-inch. Brush the remaining oil on the cut surface of each the garlic bulb.
5. Put the prepared lamb roast in the roasting pan with the garlic bulbs. Insert a meat thermometer in the center of roast and set to 140°F for medium-rare. Place in the oven and roast for about 80-85 minutes, or until the lamb is done to your preferred doneness.
6. When done, remove the lamb from the oven and let rest at least 10 minutes before carving.
7. To serve, place 2 slices of lamb of approximately ¼-inch thick on serving plates. If desired, squish a little of the garlic bulbs directly over the lamb with some of the pan juices (skim the fat first)
8. Serve with your favorite steamed vegetables.

Nutritional Information:
Calories 298, Total Fat 12.1 g, Carbs 0.3 g, Protein 40.6 g

Jalapenos Garlic Macaroni Chili Turkey

Serves: 8, **SmartPoints: 8**

Ingredients:

- 2 teaspoon chili powder
- 1 teaspoon garlic powder
- 1 teaspoon ground coriander
- 1 teaspoon onion powder
- 1 teaspoon cumin
- ¼ teaspoon salt
- 1 tablespoon olive oil
- 1 pound ground turkey
- 3 cups beef broth
- 1 (10 ounce) can tomatoes with green chilies, diced
- 2 cups dry whole wheat elbow pasta
- ½ cup low fat milk
- 4 ounces cream cheese
- 1 cup cheddar cheese, shredded
- ½ cup pickled jalapenos, chopped

Directions:

1. In a small bowl, mix together the chili powder, garlic powder, ground coriander, onion powder, chili powder, cumin, and salt.
2. In a medium saucepan, heat the olive oil on medium-high. Add the turkey and cook until it turns color. Add the spices, mix them in, and allow the mixture to cook for a further 1 or 2 minutes. Stir in the beef broth, diced tomatoes, and dry pasta. Cover the pot and cook for about 8 to 10 minutes.
3. Before the pasta finish cooking, poor the milk in a pot and place it over low heat. When the milk is warm and steamy, mix in the cheese cream until it melts. The shredded cheese can then be added to the milk. Stir until it melts.
4. Empty the cheese sauce into the pasta blend and mix until the pasta is equally covered. Blend in the pickled jalapenos. Give it a taste and add more salt if necessary. Serve hot.

Nutritional Information:
Calories 322, Total Fat 15.0 g, Carbohydrate 20.3 g, Protein 20.0 g

Sesame Oregano Grilled Salmon Kebabs

Serves: 2

Smart points: 5

Ingredients:

- ¾ pound wild salmon fillet, skinless, chopped into 1 inch pieces
- ½ teaspoon ground cumin
- 1 tablespoon fresh oregano, chopped
- ¼ teaspoon red pepper flakes
- 1 teaspoon sesame seeds
- 1 lemon sliced into thin rounds
- Kosher salt to taste
- Olive oil cooking spray
- 8 bamboo skewers soaked in water for an hour

Directions:

1. Preheat the grill to medium heat. Spray the grill grates with cooking spray.
2. Mix together in a bowl, cumin, red pepper, sesame and oregano and set aside.
3. Thread the salmon on to the skewers with the lemon slices in between.
4. Place the skewers on the grill and grill until the fish turns opaque.
5. Serve hot.

Nutritional Information: Calories: 267, Carbohydrate – 7 g, Fat – 11 g, Protein – 35 g

Delight Chicken Stroganoff

Serves: 3, **Smart points: 7**
Ingredients:
- 5.5 ounces 98% fat free cream of chicken soup or cream of mushroom soup
- 2/3 ounce onion soup mix
- ½ pound frozen chicken breast, skinless
- 8 ounces fat free sour cream

Directions:
1. Place the chicken at the bottom of the slow cooker. Mix together rest of the ingredients in a bowl and pour over and around the chicken.
2. Cover and cook on 'Low' for 6-7 hours.

Nutritional Information: Calories: 216, Carbohydrate – 15 g, Fat – 8 g, Protein – 20 g,

Raisin Grilled Chicken Salad

Serves: 4 , **SmartPoints: 6**
Ingredients:
- ¼ cup mayonnaise (low-fat)
- 1 teaspoon curry powder
- 2 teaspoons water
- 4 ounces or 1 cup rotisserie chicken, preferably lemon herb flavor, chopped
- ¾ cup apple, chopped
- ⅓ cup celery, diced
- 3 tablespoons raisins
- ⅛ teaspoon salt

Directions:
1. In a medium-sized bowl, combine the mayonnaise, curry powder, and water. Stir with a whisk until well blended.
2. Add the chopped chicken, celery, raisins, chopped apple, and salt. Stir the ingredients so they get combined well. Cover the salad and chill in the fridge. Serve in a lettuce wrap, with bread, or on its own.

Nutritional Information:
Calories 222, Total Fat 5.4 g, Carbohydrate 26.9 g, , Protein 23.0 g

Carrots Scallion Chicken Fried Rice

Serves: 4

SmartPoints: 4

Ingredients:

- 4 large egg whites
- 12 ounces boneless, skinless chicken breast, cut in ½-inch pieces
- ½ cup carrot, diced
- ½ cup scallion (green and white parts), chopped
- 2 garlic cloves, minced
- ½ cup frozen green peas, thawed
- 2 cups cooked brown rice, hot
- 3 tablespoons soy sauce (low-sodium)

Directions:

1. Coat a large, nonstick skillet with cooking spray, and set it over medium-high heat.

2. Add the egg whites and stir frequently as you cook, until they are scrambled, about 3-5 minutes. Place the eggs on a plate and set them aside.

3. Remove the pan from the heat and coat it again with cooking spray and place it over medium-high heat.

4. Add the chicken and carrots and sauté for about 5 minutes or until the chicken is golden brown. Check that the chicken is cooked through before adding the other ingredients.

5. When the chicken is ready, add the chopped scallions, minced garlic, peas, cooked brown rice, the egg whites, and soy sauce. Stir until the ingredients have combined well and continue cooking until all the ingredients are well heated.

6. Serve and enjoy.

Nutritional Information:

Calories 178, Total Fat 2.0 g Carbohydrate 21.0 g, Protein 18.0 g

Cilantro Parsley Pork Chops with Salsa

Serves: 4, **SmartPoints:4**

Ingredients:

- 4 ounces boneless pork loin chops (lean), trimmed
- Cooking spray
- ⅓ cup salsa
- 2 tablespoons lime juice, freshly squeezed
- ¼ cup fresh cilantro or parsley, chopped

Directions:

1. Place the chops on a flat surface and press each one of them with the palm of your hand to flatten them slightly.

2. Coat a large, nonstick skillet with cooking spray. Place it over high heat until the oil becomes hot. Add the chops to the skillet and cook each side for 1 minute, or until they are colored medium-brown. Reduce the heat to medium-low.

3. Mix the salsa and the fresh lime juice together and pour the mixture over the chops. Simmer, uncovered for about 8 minutes or until the chops are cooked through.

4. Garnish the chops with chopped cilantro or parsley (if desired). Serve.

Nutritional Information:

Calories 184, Total Fat 8.0 g Carbohydrate 2.0 g, Protein 25.0 g

Delicious Roasted Broccoli Balsamic Tenderlion

Serves 4, **SmartPoints:7**

Ingredients

- 1 pork tenderloin, about 1 pound
- Salt and freshly ground black pepper
- 2 bunches broccoli rabe (about 1 pound), trimmed

- Cooking spray
- 2 tablespoons olive oil, divided
- 2 tablespoons balsamic vinegar

Directions

1. Preheat oven to the broil setting and set oven rack to the upper-middle position. Line a baking sheet with parchment paper and lightly spray with cooking spray.

2. Trim the pork tenderloin from all visible fat and cut into 8 even slices. Season with salt and pepper on both sides.

3. Place broccoli rabe on the baking sheet. Spray lightly with cooking spray. Place in the oven under the broiler for 6-10 minutes until tender and golden brown. Turn the broccoli rabe over halfway through the cooking, about 4-5 minutes.

4. Warm 1 tablespoon of olive oil in a large heavy bottomed sauté pan like a cast iron over medium-high heat. Fry the pork for 8-10 minutes, turning halfway or until cooked your preferred doneness. Take the pan off the heat and remove the pork to a serving plate. Cover lightly with foil to keep warm.

5. Deglaze the pan with the balsamic vinegar and remaining 1 tablespoon of olive oil. Whisk the bottom of the pan to release the browned bits of flavors into the sauce. Season to taste with salt and pepper.

6. To serve, place 2 slices of the pork tenderloin with a quarter of the broccoli rabe on a serving plate. Pour a quarter of the sauce over the meat and vegetables and serve.

Nutritional Information:

Calories 317, Total Fat 16.1 g Carbohydrate 3.8 g, Protein 36.2 g

Garlic Sweet & Sour Chicken

Serves: 2, **Smart points: 7**

Ingredients:
- ½ pound chicken breast, skinless, boneless
- ¼ teaspoon onion powder
- ¼ teaspoon garlic powder
- 2.5 ounces sweet and sour sauce
- 4 ounces canned pineapple chunks with 2-3 tablespoons of its juice
- 8 ounces stir fry vegetables
- ½ tablespoon brown sugar
- Cooking spray

Directions:
1. Spray the inside of the crock-pot with cooking spray.
2. Place the chicken in the crock-pot. Season the chicken with garlic powder and onion powder,
3. Mix together rest of the ingredients except vegetables and pour over the chicken.
4. Cover and cook on 'Low' for 6-7 hours.

Nutritional Information: Calories: 206, Carbohydrate – 19 g, Fat – 3 g, Protein – 25 g,

Weekend Treat Beef Burgundy

Serves: 3, **Smart points: 13**

Ingredients:
- 1 pound round steak, trimmed of fat, chopped into bite size pieces
- 1 clove garlic, minced
- 1 tablespoon tomato paste
- 1 medium onion, sliced
- 8 ounces frozen small whole onions, thawed, drained

- 5 ounces condensed beef broth, undiluted
- 3 tablespoons all purpose flour
- ¼ cup red wine
- 4 ounces fresh mushrooms sliced
- ¼ teaspoon dried thyme
- ½ teaspoon salt or to taste
- 1 bay leaf
- Pepper to taste
- 1 ½ cups medium egg noodles, cook according to the instructions on the package
- Cooking spray

Directions:

1. Place a skillet over medium heat. Spray with cooking spray. Add beef and sauté until brown. Transfer into the slow cooker.
2. Spray again with cooking spray. Add sliced onions and garlic and sauté until translucent. Add flour and sauté for about a minute.
3. Add broth, wine and tomato paste. Stir constantly until thick. Add whole onions, mushrooms, bay leaf, thyme, pepper and salt and stir. Transfer into the instant pot.
4. Cover and cook on 'High' for an hour. Then switch to 'Low' and cook for 4 ½ hours.
5. When done, discard the bay leaf.
6. Divide the egg noodles in 3 bowls. Ladle beef over it and serve.

Nutritional Information: Calories: 488, Carbohydrate – 38.1 g, , Fat – 17 g, Protein – 41.3 g

Tasty Turkey Cheeseburger & Broccoli Slaw

Cooking time: 15 minutes, Serves: 10
Smart points: 8

Ingredients:
- 2 ½ pounds 93% lean ground turkey
- 3 cups broccoli slaw
- 1 1/3 cups carrots, grated
- ½ cup blue cheese dressing
- 2 cloves garlic, grated
- ½ cup seasoned whole wheat breadcrumbs
- 1 tablespoon red onion, grated
- Salt to taste
- Freshly ground pepper to taste
- ½ cup hot sauce or to taste
- 10 slices low fat cheddar
- Cooking spray
- 10 whole wheat burger buns, split

Directions:
1. Mix together in a bowl, turkey, breadcrumbs, carrots, onion, garlic, salt, pepper and hot sauce. Divide into 10 portions and shape each portion into a patty.
2. Mix together in a bowl, broccoli slaw and blue cheese dressing and set aside.
3. Place a skillet over high heat. Spray with cooking spray. Place 2-3 patties at a time.
4. Lower heat to medium low. Cook until the bottom side is golden brown. Flip sides and cook the other side too. Cook the burgers in batches.
5. Toast the burger buns. Place a patty over each bun. Top with cheese and broccoli slaw and serve.

Nutritional Information: Calories: 358, Carbohydrate – 22.7 g, Fat – 15 g, Protein – 38.3 g

Coriander Jalapenos Sour Spicy Beef

Makes: 6 servings, **SmartPoints: 4**

Ingredients

- 2 lbs. top beef eye round (lean, trimmed of fat)
- 1 sweet onion (diced)
- 2 garlic cloves (sliced)
- 1 red bell pepper (diced)
- 2 jalapenos
- ¼ cup beef broth (low-sodium)
- 1 cup canned diced tomatoes with juice
- 1 tablespoon coconut aminos
- 2 tablespoon fresh lime juice
- ½ teaspoon cumin
- ¼ teaspoon oregano
- ¼ teaspoon coriander

Directions:

- Season the beef with salt and pepper and place it in a slow cooker.
- Add the rest of the ingredients to the slow cooker.
- Leave to cook for 8 hours on low.
- Slice and serve.

Nutritional information: Calories: 233; Total Fat: 5 g; Carbohydrates: 8 g; Proteins: 36 g

Ginger Sesame Chicken

Serves: 4, **SmartPoints: 6**

Ingredients:

- 1 pound boneless, skinless chicken breast
- 2 teaspoons coconut oil
- ½ teaspoon salt
- 1 teaspoon coarse ground black pepper
- ½ teaspoon cayenne powder
- 1 tablespoon freshly grated ginger

- 2 tablespoons honey
- ¼ cup soy sauce
- 2 teaspoons sesame oil
- 1 tablespoon sesame seeds, toasted (optional)
- Fresh lemongrass for garnish, optional
- Cooked rice for serving (optional)

Directions:

1. Using a meat mallet, flatten the chicken until it is approximately ¼ inch thick.

2. Melt the coconut oil in a skillet over medium heat.

3. Season the chicken with salt, black pepper, and cayenne powder. Cook the chicken in the skillet for 4-5 minutes per side, or until it is no longer pink in the center.

4. In a small bowl, combine the fresh ginger, honey, soy sauce, and sesame oil. Mix well and pour the sauce over the chicken.

5. Continue cooking, just until the liquid begins to bubble, approximately 1-2 minutes.

6. Remove from the heat and serve warm, garnished with sesame seeds and lemongrass, if desired.

Nutritional Information: Calories 210, Fat 7.5 g, Carbohydrate 8.9 g, Protein 25.9 g

Tomato Lime Beef Curry

Makes: 4 servings

SmartPoints: 4

Ingredients

- 1 lb. ground beef (95% lean)
- 1 leek (thinly sliced)
- 2 garlic cloves (minced)
- 1 teaspoon fresh ginger (raw)
- 1 tablespoon red curry paste
- 1 1/2 cups canned tomato sauce
- 1 teaspoon lime zest
- 1 tablespoon coconut aminos

- ½ cup canned light coconut milk
- 2 teaspoon lime juice

Directions:

•	Brown the beef in a skillet and then transfer it to a slow cooker.

•	Add the rest of the ingredients to the slow cooker except the coconut milk and lime juice.

•	Leave to cook for 4 hours on low.

•	Add the lime juice and coconut milk, stir and cook for another 15 minutes.

Nutritional information:

Calories: 213; Total Fat: 8 g; Carbohydrates: 10 g; Proteins: 26 g

Chapter 4 Weight Watchers Seafood

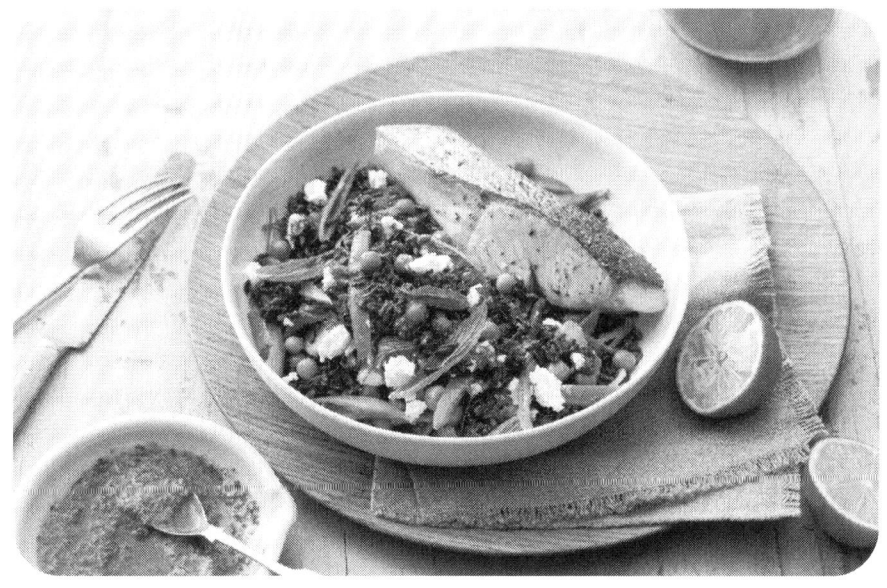

Lemon Dijon Whitefish

Serves: 4, **SmartPoints: 1**

Ingredients:
- 1 pound whitefish fillets
- Cooking spray
- 2 tablespoons Dijon mustard
- 1 teaspoon prepared horseradish
- 1 tablespoon fresh lemon juice
- 1 teaspoon salt
- 1 teaspoon black pepper
- 1 lemon, sliced

Directions:
1. Preheat the oven to 450°F and spray a 9x9 or larger baking dish with cooking spray.
2. In a bowl, combine the Dijon mustard, horseradish, and lemon juice.
3. Brush each whitefish fillet with the Dijon mixture, season with salt and pepper as desired, and then place it in the baking dish.
4. Place the lemon slices over the top of the fish.
5. Place the fish in the oven and bake for 15 minutes, or until the fish is cooked through and flakey.

Nutritional Information: Calories 99, Total Fat 1.0 g, Carbohydrate 0.4 g, Protein 20.0 g

Ginger Chili Salmon

Makes: 5 servings, **SmartPoints: 5**

Ingredients
- 30 oz. coho salmon fillets (skinless)
- ¼ teaspoon salt
- ¼ teaspoon pepper
- ¼ teaspoon smoked paprika
- ¼ teaspoon ground ginger
- ¾ teaspoon ground cumin
- 2 ½ teaspoon olive oil
- 2 ½ teaspoon chili powder

Directions:
- Mix all the dry spices in a bowl.

- Spray the salmon with cooking spray and rub the spice mixture into it.
- Heat oil in a pan and cook the salmon fillets in it for 4-5 minutes per side.

Nutritional information: Calories: 274; Total Fat: 12 g; Carbohydrates: 1 g; Proteins: 37 g

Dill Coriander Cucumber Salmon

Serves: 4, **SmartPoints: 3**

Ingredients:

- 1 pound salmon steaks
- ½ cup plain low fat Greek yogurt
- ½ cup cucumber, peeled and finely diced
- 1 tablespoon fresh dill, chopped
- ½ teaspoon salt
- 1 teaspoon black pepper
- 1 tablespoon olive oil or cooking spray
- ½ teaspoon ground coriander
- 1 teaspoon fresh lemon juice

Directions:

1. Prepare a stovetop grill over medium heat.
2. In a bowl combine the low fat Greek yogurt, cucumber, dill and a pinch of the salt and black pepper. Mix well and place in the refrigerator until ready to serve.
3. Brush the salmon steaks with olive oil or spray a light coat of cooking spray. Season the salmon with the remaining salt, black pepper, coriander, and lemon juice.
4. Place the salmon steaks on the grill, and cook 12-15 minutes, depending on thickness, turning once about halfway through, until the salmon is flakey in the center.
5. Remove from the heat and serve with a dollop of cucumber sauce.

Nutritional Information:

Calories 186, Total Fat 5.0 g, Carbohydrate 2.9 g, Protein 30.6 g

Cherry Tomato Asparagus Lobster Salad

Makes: 2 servings, **SmartPoints: 5**

Ingredients
- 8 oz. lobster (cooked, chopped)
- 3 ½ cups asparagus (chopped, steamed)
- 2 tablespoon lemon juice
- 4 teaspoons extra-virgin olive oil
- ¼ teaspoon kosher salt
- Black pepper to taste
- ½ cup cherry tomatoes (halved)
- 1 basil leaf (chopped)
- 2 tablespoon red onion (diced)

Directions:
- Whisk together the lemon juice, salt, pepper and oil in a bowl.
- Toss together the rest of the ingredients in a salad bowl.
- Pour the dressing over and toss again.

Nutritional information:
Calories: 247; Total Fat: 10.5 g; Carbohydrates: 14 g; Proteins: 27 g

Delicious Coconut Salmon

Makes: 5 servings, **SmartPoints: 5**

Ingredients
- 30 oz. salmon (skinless, boneless)
- 1/3 cup unsweetened coconut (shredded)
- 2 egg whites (whisked)
- Salt and pepper to taste

Directions:
- Season the salmon with salt and pepper.
- Dip the salmon into the egg and then dredge it with the coconut.
- Arrange the fish on a wire rack placed over a baking dish.
- Bake for 10-12 minutes in an oven preheated to 400 degrees Fahrenheit.

Nutritional information:

Calories: 293; Total Fat: 14 g; Carbohydrates: 1 g; Proteins: 39 g

Spices Honey Shrimp Baked

Serves: 4
SmartPoints: 3

Ingredients:
- Olive oil cooking spray
- 1 tablespoon honey
- 2 teaspoons creole seasoning
- 2 teaspoons parsley, dried
- 1 teaspoon olive oil
- 2 tablespoons lemon juice, freshly squeezed
- 2 teaspoons soy sauce (low-sodium)
- 1 pound large shrimp, peeled

Directions:
1. Preheat the oven to 450°F. Coat an 11x7 baking dish with the olive oil spray.
2. In the baking dish, combine the honey, creole seasoning, dried parsley, olive oil, lemon juice, and soy sauce and stir well so that all the ingredients have combined well.
3. Add the shrimp to the mixture and toss it to coat.
4. Bake the coated shrimp for about 8 minutes, or until turns pink, but ensure you keep stirring from time to time. Remove from the oven and serve.

Nutritional Information:
Calories 111, Total Fat 2.0 g, Carbohydrate 6.0 g, Protein 16.0 g

Simple Tuna Salad

Serves: 4

SmartPoints: 4

Ingredients:
- ½ pound tuna, canned or cooked and flaked
- 1 cup artichoke hearts, quartered
- 1 cup red bell pepper, chopped
- 1 cup cherry tomatoes, quartered
- 1 tablespoon lemon juice
- 2 tablespoons olive oil
- 1 teaspoon salt
- 1 teaspoon black pepper
- ½ teaspoon oregano
- ½ cup fresh parsley, chopped (optional)
- Leaf lettuce for serving (optional)

Directions:
1. In a bowl, combine the tuna, artichoke hearts, red bell pepper, and tomatoes. Toss to mix.
2. Drizzle the salad with lemon juice and olive oil, then season with salt, black pepper, and oregano. Add the fresh parsley last, and toss gently to mix.
3. Cover and refrigerate for at least 30 minutes before serving.
4. Serve on a bed of leaf lettuce, if desired.

Nutritional Information:
Calories 163, Total Fat 7.8 g, Carbohydrate 5.0 g, Protein 18.0 g

Ginger Honey Glazed Salmon

Serves: 4, **SmartPoints: 4**

Ingredients:
- 4 pieces salmon fillet
- 3 tablespoons rice wine (sweet)
- 1 tablespoon honey
- 1 tablespoon rice vinegar, seasoned
- 1 tablespoon soy sauce
- 1 teaspoon ginger, minced
- ¼ cup scallions, thinly sliced
- Salt and pepper to taste
- Cooking spray

Directions:
1. In a small saucepan, mix the sweet wine, honey, vinegar, soy sauce, and ginger. Bring them to a boil over medium-high heat to make the sauce. Cook the sauce while stirring regularly for about 5 minutes, until it has thickened and the flavors have blended well. Remove it from the heat and then cover it with a lid to keep it warm.
2. In the meantime, sprinkle the salmon with salt and pepper and spray a large nonstick skillet with the vegetable oil spray. Set it over high heat. Add the salmon fillet pieces and cook for about 4 minutes on each side, or until the fish is browned. Turn the fillet once halfway through. Use a spoon to spread the sauce over the fish and sprinkle with the scallions. Serve hot.

Nutritional Information:
Calories 180, Total Fat 5.0 g, Carbohydrate 5.9 g, Protein 23.7 g

Spinach Tomato Shrimp Pasta

Serves: 4

SmartPoints: 8

Ingredients:

- 8 ounces angel hair (vermicelli) pasta, cooked
- ½ cup onion, diced
- 2 cups heirloom tomatoes, chopped
- 1 pound shrimp, cleaned and deveined
- 6 cups fresh spinach, torn
- 1 tablespoon olive oil
- 1 teaspoon salt
- 1 teaspoon black pepper
- 1 teaspoon crushed red pepper flakes

Directions:

1. Pour the olive oil in a large skillet over medium heat.
2. Place the onion in the skillet and sauté for 2-3 minutes.
3. Add the tomatoes and cook for an additional 2 minutes.
4. Add the shrimp to the skillet, and cook for 5 minutes, stirring frequently. The shrimp should turn pink.
5. Place the spinach in the skillet with the other ingredients and cook until wilted, approximately 1-2 minutes.
6. Add the cooked pasta to the skillet and toss to mix. Reduce the heat to low and cook until the pasta is heated through, approximately 2-4 minutes. Remove from the heat and serve immediately.

Nutritional Information: Calories 357, Total Fat 3.5 g, Carbohydrate 50g, Protein 32.3 g

Yummy Tuna Salad & Pasta

Serves: 6

SmartPoints: 5

Ingredients:

- 6 ounces pasta
- 1 (12 ounce) can tuna, drained
- ¼ cup celery, diced
- ½ cup cherry tomatoes cut in halves
- ½ cup yellow bell pepper, cut into strips
- ¾ cup salsa, (low-salt)
- ½ cup mayonnaise (low-fat)
- ½ teaspoon red pepper, ground
- 2 tablespoons scallions, sliced

Directions:

1. Start by cooking the pasta according to the package instructions, but omit the fat and salt.
2. Drain the pasta and rinse it with cold water.
3. In a large bowl, mix together the pasta, tuna, celery, cherry tomatoes, and sliced bell pepper until everything has combined well.
4. In a small bowl, mix together the salsa, mayonnaise, and ground red pepper until they have combined well. Add the dressing to the pasta mixture and toss. Cover and chill. Sprinkle the mixture with scallions and serve.

Nutritional Information: Calories 194, Total Fat 2.0 g Carbohydrate 25.0 g, Protein 18.0 g

Asian Style Sesame Glazed Salmon

Serves: 4
SmartPoints: 3

Ingredients:
- 1 pound salmon steaks
- Cooking spray
- 2 tablespoons soy sauce
- 1 tablespoon rice vinegar
- 1 tablespoon shallots, diced
- ½ teaspoon salt
- 1 teaspoon black pepper
- 1 tablespoon toasted sesame seeds

Directions:
1. Spray a skillet with the cooking spray and heat it over medium high.
2. In a bowl, combine the soy sauce, rice vinegar and shallots. Whisk until blended.
3. Season the salmon with salt and black pepper and then brush each steak with the glaze.
4. Reduce the heat of the skillet to medium and place the salmon in the pan, skin side down (if the skin is still attached).
5. Cook for 5-7 minutes per side, or until the salmon is cooked through.
6. Remove from the skillet and sprinkle with toasted sesame seeds before serving.

Nutritional Information: Calories 186, Total Fat 6.1 g, Carbohydrate 1.1 g, Protein 29.9 g

Coconut Curry Scallops

Serves: 4

SmartPoints: 8

Ingredients:
- 1 pound scallops
- Cooking spray
- 1 cup onion, thinly sliced
- 1 cup red bell pepper, thinly sliced
- 1 teaspoon salt
- 1 teaspoon black pepper
- 1 ½ cups unsweetened coconut milk
- 1 tablespoon curry powder
- Fresh cilantro for garnish (optional)
- Cooked rice for serving (optional)

Directions:

1. Preheat the oven to 375°F, and lightly spray an 8x8 or larger baking dish.
2. Place the onion and red bell pepper in the baking dish, followed by the scallops.
3. Season the scallops with salt and black pepper.
4. Combine the coconut milk with the curry powder and pour it over the scallops.
5. Place the baking dish in the oven and bake for 15 minutes, or until the scallops are cooked through.
6. Remove it from the oven and let it rest for 3-5 minutes before serving.
7. Garnish with fresh cilantro and serve with cooked rice, if desired.

Nutritional Information:

Calories 249, Total Fat 16.9 g, Carbohydrate 10.7 g, Protein 25.8 g

Yummy Ginger Soy Sauce Salmon

Serves: 6

SmartPoints: 5

Ingredients:

- 6 fillets fresh salmon, skinned
- ⅓ cup soy sauce
- ¼ cup brown sugar
- 2 garlic cloves, minced
- 2 teaspoon fresh ginger, minced

Directions:

1. Prepare the marinade in advance by combining soy sauce, brown sugar, ginger, and garlic together in a small bowl. Place the salmon fillets in a large resealable bag and pour in the marinade. Turn the bag to coat the salmon, and refrigerate.

2. Turn the fish from time to time so the marinade can cover it all. In the meantime, preheat the oven to 425°F.

3. Remove the fish from the fridge and seal it in a square of aluminum foil. Place it on a baking sheet and put it in the oven.

4. Cook for 15 minutes, or until the salmon is properly cooked. You'll know it has cooked through when it flakes easily when pressed with a fork. Serve immediately and enjoy.

Nutritional Information: Calories 192.0, Total Fat 7.0 g, Carbohydrate 7.0 g, Protein 23.0 g

Romaine Watermelon Salad & Shrimp

Serves: 4   **SmartPoints: 7**

Ingredients:

For the shrimp:
- 10 ounces large shrimp, shelled and deveined
- 1 garlic clove, crushed to a paste
- Salt to taste (seasoned)

For dressing:
- 1 tablespoon shallots, chopped
- 1 teaspoon water
- 2 ½ tablespoons golden balsamic vinegar
- ⅛ teaspoon kosher salt
- Pinch of black pepper
- 2 tablespoons extra-virgin olive oil

For salad:
- 8 cups romaine, chopped
- 4 cups watermelon, diced
- 4 ounces soft goat cheese

Directions:

1. Take a small bowl and mix shallots, water, vinegar, salt, and pepper. Add olive oil little by little stirring until it has combined well. Season the shrimp with seasoned salt, and then add the garlic, mixing it in. You may thread the shrimp onto pre-soaked skewers. Light the grill (or use an indoor grill pan if you are not using skewers) on medium to medium-high heat. Grill each side of the shrimp for about 1 or 2 minutes. Set them aside when ready. In a large bowl, toss the romaine with the dressing. Divide it on 4 plates. Top with watermelon, goat cheese, and the shrimp. Enjoy.

Nutritional Information: Calories 293, Total Fat 18.0 g, Carbohydrate 12.0 g, Protein 22.0 g

Parsley Garlic Pasta Shrimp

Serves: 1

SmartPoints: 7

Ingredients:
- ¼ cup chopped onions
- 2 garlic cloves, chopped
- 1 teaspoon olive oil
- 2 tablespoons white wine
- ½ cup cooked shrimp
- Fresh parsley, to taste
- 1 cup whole wheat pasta, cooked
- 1 tablespoon Parmesan cheese, grated
- Black pepper, coarsely ground

Directions:
1. Sauté the onions and garlic in a nonstick skillet with the olive oil.
2. Add the white wine and reduce the heat.
3. Stir in the shrimp and parsley, and cook until the shrimp is warmed through.
4. Add the cooked pasta and stir until all the pasta has been coated. Add the cheese and pepper. Serve and enjoy. You can serve with a green salad to enrich it and make the meal very satisfying.

Nutritional Information:
Calories 415, Total Fat 8.5 g, Carbohydrate 46.7 g, Protein 35.1 g

Chapter 5: Weight Watchers Desserts Recipes

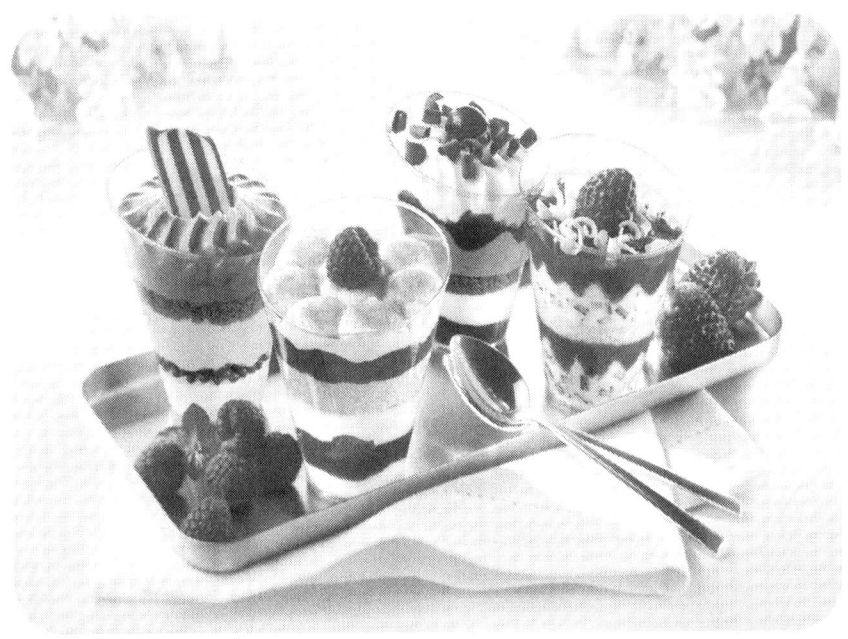

Chocolate Cheesecake Cups

Serves: 6

Smart points: 3

Ingredients:
- 1 small egg
- ½ ounce semisweet baking chocolate + extra shavings to garnish
- 2 tablespoons sugar
- 2 ounces 1/3 less fat cream cheese, softened
- 2 tablespoons light sour cream

Directions:
1. Line mini muffin cups with cupcake liners.
2. Melt the chocolate either in a microwave or in a double boiler.
3. Add cream cheese and sugar to a bow. Beat with a hand mixer. Add sour cream and continue beating until smooth.
4. Add egg and fold gently with a spoon. Add melted chocolate and stir until well combined.
5. Place about 2 tablespoons of the mixture in each muffin cup.
6. Bake in a preheated oven at 225° F for about 50 minutes.
7. Once baked, let it remain in the oven for about 30 minutes.
8. Remove from the oven and cool completely.
9. Chill for a few hours. Sprinkle the chocolate shavings over it and serve.

Nutrition Information: Calories: 65, Carbohydrate – 6 g, Fat – 4 g, Protein – 1.5 g

Raspberry Coconut Chia Pudding

Serves: 4, **Smart points: 5, Ingredients:**
- 1 cup light coconut milk
- 2 cups raspberries
- 4 tablespoons chia seeds
- 1 cup almond coconut milk, unsweetened
- 2 tablespoons shredded coconut, sweetened
- 2 teaspoons lime zest
- 2 teaspoons lime juice
- 15-16 drops stevia drops or to taste

Directions:
1. Retain half the raspberries and mix the remaining raspberries with rest of the ingredients in a bowl. Cover and chill for 5-6 hours.
2. Divide the mixture into 4 serving bowls. Divide the raspberries that were set-aside over it and serve.

Nutrition Information: Calories: 157, Carbohydrate – 15 g, Fat – 10 g, Protein – 4 g

Delicious Pumpkin Pudding

Serves: 2, **SmartPoints: 3**
Ingredients:
- 1 ½ cups skim milk
- 1 (15 ounce) can pure pumpkin
- ½ box instant vanilla pudding (sugar free and fat free)
- 1 tablespoon ground allspice
- 1 tablespoon cinnamon
- Add brown sugar to taste

Directions:
1. To make thick pumpkin, combine skim milk and pumpkin in a pan and stir. Add the instant pudding and combine.
2. Add the remaining ingredients and stir. Add more seasonings to taste if desired. Heat and stir occasionally until the soup is warm. Enjoy.

Nutritional Information:

Calories 163, Total Fat 0.9 g, Carbohydrate 30.8 g, Protein 9.5 g

Walnut Dark Chocolate Clusters

Serves: 10, **Smart points: 2**

Ingredients:

- 10 pecan halves
- 10 almonds
- 10 walnut halves
- Sea salt as required
- ½ package Ghirardelli dark chocolate melting wafers

Directions:

1. Melt the chocolate either in a double boiler or in a microwave.
2. Pick a walnut with a fork and dip into the melted chocolate. Shake off the excess chocolate and place on a tray lined with wax paper. Repeat this procedure with the pecan and place the dipped pecan over the walnut. Finally repeat this procedure with the almond and place over the pecan. This makes one cluster. Sprinkle a few grains of salt over it.
3. Repeat the above process with the remaining nuts and chocolate. Makes 10 clusters in all.

Nutrition Information: Calories: 54, Carbohydrate – 3 g, Fat – 5 g, Protein – 1 g

Simple Truffles

Yields 24, 2 truffles per serving, **SmartPoints: 2**

Ingredients:

- 1 cup powdered sugar
- ½ cup cocoa, unsweetened
- ½ cup fat-free cream cheese
- ½ teaspoon vanilla extract

Directions:

1. Prepare a baking sheet with parchment paper, and sprinkle it cocoa powder.

2.	Mix all the ingredients with an electric mixer. Use a rounded teaspoon to drop the mixture onto the sheet.
3.	Roll the mixture into balls and put in the refrigerator.
Nutritional Information:
Calories 36, Total Fat 0 g, Carbohydrate 6.8 g, Protein 0.8 g

Fruit Parfaits Candy Corn

Serves: 4, **Smart points: 3**
Ingredients:
For the lighter whipped topping:
- ¼ cup heavy whipping cream, chilled
- ¼ cup fat free plain Greek yogurt
- 1 tablespoon sugar
- ¼ teaspoon vanilla

For parfaits:
- 1 1/3 cups jarred mandarin oranges, drained
- 1 1/3 cups diced pineapple (canned or fresh)

Directions:
1.	Add sugar, vanilla, and cream into a bowl and beat with a chilled hand beater until stiff peaks are formed.
2.	Add yogurt and fold.
3.	Layer in parfait glasses using mandarin oranges, pineapple and whipped cream.
4.	Chill for a while and serve.
Nutrition Information: Calories: 151, Carbohydrate – 23 g, Fat – 6 g, Protein – 3 g

Frozen Pineapple Berry Dessert

Serves: 24, **SmartPoints: 1**
Ingredients:
1 can whole berry cranberry sauce
1 can pineapplc, crushed
1 container whipped topping (fat free)
1/4 cup walnuts, chopped

Directions:
1.	Mix all the ingredients together and combine well. Divide the mixture into 24 cupcake pans with liners. Freeze. Remove the frozen desserts and place them in a plastic bag and

then store in the freezer. Enjoy one whenever you want something sweet and cold.

Nutritional Information:

Calories 63, Total Fat 0.8 g, Carbohydrate 13.4 g, Protein 0.1 g

Vanilla Cranberry Coconut Macaroons

Serves: 12, 2 macaroons per serving

SmartPoints: 2

Ingredients:

- 2 egg whites (large size)
- ¼ teaspoon salt
- ⅓ cup sugar
- 1 cup sweetened flaked coconut
- ½ cup dried cranberries
- 2 tablespoons all-purpose flour
- ½ teaspoon vanilla extract
- Cooking spray

Directions:

1. Preheat the oven to 325°F, and coat 2 cooking sheets with vegetable oil spray, or line them with parchment paper.

2. In a medium bowl, combine the egg whites and salt. Use an electric mixer to beat at low speed for about 1 minute, until the egg whites foam.

3. Gradually add the sugar as you increase the mixer speed for about 5 to 7 minutes.

4. Fold in the remaining ingredients. Drop the batter using a tablespoon onto a cookie sheet. Bake for about 15 minutes or until the macaroons become light golden brown. Remove from the oven and serve.

Nutritional Information:

Calories 68. Total Fat 3.0 g Carbohydrate 10.0 g, Protein 1.0 g

Nutmeg Pumpkin Cheesecake

Serves: 8, **Smart points: 3**

Ingredients:
- 0.75 ounces chocolate Graham crackers
- ¼ cup pure canned pumpkin
- 2 ounces 1/3 fat cream cheese, softened
- ½ teaspoon vanilla extract
- ½ teaspoon pumpkin pie spice
- 4 ounces light whipped topping
- 1 ½ tablespoons dark brown sugar, unpacked
- 1/8 teaspoon ground cinnamon
- 1/8 teaspoon ground nutmeg

Directions:
1. Place the crackers in a food processor and pulse until crumb like texture is formed. Set aside for a while.
2. Add cream cheese into a bowl and beat with an electric mixer until smooth.
3. Add vanilla, sugar, pumpkin, pumpkin pie spice, cinnamon and nutmeg and beat until smooth and creamy.
4. Add about 2.5 ounces of the whipped topping and mix well. Transfer into a piping bag. Take 8 shot glasses. Sprinkle about ½ teaspoon of cracker crumbs at the bottom of each shot glass. Pipe out some of the pumpkin mixture over it. Dot with a little whipped topping (about a teaspoon). Repeat the above layer once. Finally top with some crumbs.
8. Chill and serve later.

Nutrition Information: Calories: 78, Carbohydrate – 11.6 g, Fat – 4.2 g, Protein – 1 g

Vanilla Cupcake Brownies

Serves: 12

SmartPoints: 2

Ingredients:

- ¾ cup all-purpose flour
- ½ cup sugar, preferably brown
- 3 tablespoons cocoa, unsweetened
- ½ teaspoon baking soda
- ¼ teaspoon salt
- ½ cup water
- ¼ cup applesauce, unsweetened
- 1 tablespoon brown sugar, firmly packed
- 1 ½ teaspoons margarine, melted
- ½ teaspoon vanilla extract
- ½ teaspoon cider vinegar
- Cooking spray (optional)

Directions:

1. Preheat the oven to 350°F. In a large bowl, combine the flour, brown sugar, unsweetened cocoa, baking soda, and salt. Mix well.

2. In another bowl, stir together all the other ingredients. Pour the mixture over the flour mixture and stir just until the batter is smooth.

3. Coat a nonstick muffin tin with 12 cups with vegetable oil spray, or line them with paper liners. Pour the batter into the muffin cups until they're half full.

4. Bake for 18 to 20 minutes. To ensure that the cupcakes are cooked, prick them in the center with a toothpick and if it comes out clean, they are ready. Remove them from the oven and let them stand for 5 minutes before transferring them to the rack to cool. Enjoy.

Nutritional Information:

Calories 78, Total Fat 0.7 g, Carbohydrate 17.3 g, Protein 1.1 g

Raspberry Jam Banana Roll Ups

Serves: 1, **SmartPoints: 5**

Ingredients:

- 1 6-inch whole wheat tortilla
- 1 tablespoon peanut butter (reduced-fat)
- 1 teaspoon raspberry jam (sugar-free)
- 1 teaspoon dried coconut (unsweetened), shredded
- ½ medium-sized ripe banana, sliced

Directions:

1. Lay the whole wheat tortilla on a flat surface and spread the peanut butter and jam evenly on it. Sprinkle the dried shredded coconut on top.
2. Arrange the banana pieces on the tortilla. Roll up the tortilla to enclose the banana pieces. Wrap it in a paper towel and put in the microwave on high mode for 30 to 35 seconds.
3. Remove from microwave and unwrap from the paper towel. Enjoy.

Nutritional Information:

Calories 160, Total Fat 7.0 g, Carbohydrate 25.0 g, Protein 5.0 g

Chapter 5 Conclusion

Thank you again for purchasing my book!

I hope you've enjoyed this book, I'd like to ask you for a favor, would you be kind enough to leave a review for this book on Amazon? It'd be greatly appreciated!

Thank you and good luck!
Regards
Anthony Young

Made in the USA
Middletown, DE
28 January 2018